BREAKING the AUTISM CODE

A GUIDE FOR NEW PARENTS, LYME, TOXICITY, THE GUT, AND VACCINES

By Cindy Lang Walsh

©2017 Cindy Lang Walsh

BREAKING THE AUTISM CODE

Copyright @2017 By Cindy Lang Walsh
Cover Design By Patrise Henkel
Editor: Carol Burbank

The information contained in this book has been researched over many years in the interviews I have conducted with other families and our own journey. This is not a replacement for help from a medical professional. The Author is not a doctor and the information contained herein is not considered medical advice.

Names used in the stories of this book are fictional, as the real people used in these stories do not want to be identified.

All Rights Reserved. No part of this book may be reproduced or transmitted in any form or by any means electronic or mechanical including photocopying or recording without written permission from the publisher, except for inclusion of brief passages in a review, forum or blog with reference to the book.

This book was manufactured in the U.S.A.

Publishers Catalogue
Prepared by The New Normal Press.

Walsh, Cindy Lang

ISBN 1542767156

Please visit:
Breakingtheautismcode.com

This book is dedicated to all the confused parents who are just beginning their autism journey. The Autism World is lonely. You are among family.

Special Thanks to Cindy Davis, I hope you find this book and know that I did finally finish the book we set out to write together.

Thanks to Carol Burbank who spent so many years editing and formatting to make this book the best it can be. Thanks to Patrise Henkel who designed the cover, as well as the website, and has given me great feedback along the way.

Thanks to Maria, Clay and Virginia Young, Lisa Marks Smith, and Linda Weinmaster, who have submitted their vaccine injury stories. Thanks to Jennifer and Ronnie Prine for their encouragement and support. I would also thank Amy Trail and Teresa Champion who gave me great advice and helpful tips about IEP meetings.

Thanks to Warren and Susan Levin, and Debbie McCabe and Susan Greenberg for taking care of my family and of me.

Thanks to every parent who let me interview them to talk about their kids. Thanks to my family as well, because this book took so long.

Contents

Introduction 1
    Why Is this Book Important? 3
Part 1: The Gut, The Brain and the Immune System 17
    David: The Poop Decorator 19
    Why Is the Gut Important in Autism? 28
    Joey: The Climber 35
    Other Food Issues 42
        Not Absorbing Nutrients 44
    How Do We Make the Gut Healthy Again? 47
Part 2: How Does Lyme Disease Affect Behavior and Physical Health? 49
    Pete: The Refuser 51
    Why Is Lyme Important? 57
Part 3: Toxicity: How does Environment Affect Behavior? 67
    Nathan: The Personality Changer 69
    Why Is Understanding Toxicity So Important? 79
    How Do We Make Our Children Healthy Again? 97
Part 4: Why are Vaccines So Controversial? 101
    Jacob: The Threat 103
    Frequently Asked Questions About Vaccines 110
    Vaccine Ingredients: Which Offer the Greatest Risks? 135
    Who is Vulnerable to Vaccine Injury? 141
    How Do I Get the Facts to Make an Informed Decision? 152
    Downplaying the Risk: Hiding the Liability and Risk of Vaccine Injuries 155
Part 5: Friendly Advice on Detoxification, Diets and IEP Success 169
    How to Change Your Family Diet and Support Detoxification? 171

Three Ways To Clean the Gut 173

Common Sense, Practical Ways to Detoxify 174

Common Tests 175

Behaviors 176

Tools to Track Success 181

What You Can Do In The School Setting: Advice For Team Building And Successful IEPs 183

Rules for Navigating Your IEP 187

Types of things the behavior specialist can do for you 191

Types of Things an Advocate can do for you. 192

Labels You Might Encounter at Your IEP Meeting 193

Tests Your School Might Offer to Determine the Best Services for Your Child 198

Legal Terms 203

Government Agencies 204

People Who May Work with your Child 205

Other Medical References 206

Frequent Mistakes Schools Make About Our Kids 207

Part 6: Decoding Other Behaviors Using this Guide: More Stories 213

   Introduction 215

   The Sensitive Child 217

      MICHAEL: The Empathic Child. 217

      SARAH: The Burn Patient 226

      Advice for Parents of Sensitive Children 232

   The Learning-Disabled Child 234

      DOUGLAS: Obsessed with Letters and Numbers 234

      WILLIAM: The Fumbling Child 245

      Advice To Parents with Learning-Disabled Kids 253

The Hyper Child 256
    ANDREW: The Squirmy Kid 256
    BENJAMIN: The Screamer.. 260
The Exhausted Child 264
    JUSTIN: Tired and Slow 264
    CALEB: The Snorer 270
    Advice to Parents with Exhausted Children 275
The Depressed or Angry Child 277
    KRISTEN: The Dirt Police 277
    JENNY: The Fragile Child 281
    Advice to Parents of Depressed or Angry Children 284

Part 7: Conclusion.. 287
Do Not Comply: Tell the Truth Instead 289

Part 8: APPENDICES 295
Appendix A: The Stool Chart... 297
Appendix B: Yeast Symptoms 298
Appendix C: Always Eat Organic 299
Appendix D: Ingredients That Contain MSG 300
Appendix E: Ingredients That May Contain MSG 301
Appendix F: Comparison Chart for Symptoms of MS, Lyme Disease, Fibromyalgia and CFS.. 302
Appendix G: Common Signs of Toxicity from Dr. Doris Rapp 304
Appendix H: 15 Toxic Occupations 305
Appendix I: US Mortality Rates for Polio, Smallpox, Diptheria, & Typhoid 306
Appendix J: Vaccine Information Statement vs. Vaccine Insert 307
Appendix K: 28 studies from around the world that support Dr. Wakefield's controversial findings: 308

Appendix L: Behavior Chart 310

Appendix M: State Vaccine Exemptions 312

Appendix N: Vaccines that Contain Aborted Fetal Cells
(reasons for religious exemptions) 314

Appendix O: Recommended Books 316

End Notes 318

Introduction

Why Is this Book Important?

This book is an overview of many medical issues that people on the spectrum have that can sometimes create symptoms we know as autism. Autism is multi-faceted and can take many years to understand and treat. Unfortunately, some damage cannot be undone. It takes a lifetime and extra expenses, time, and expertise to correct medical issues and control behaviors to help the child concentrate on academics. The system is set up to manage academic and social behavior, and treat the pain last, if at all. But we can't give up. We can improve our children's lives by treating medical issues to support behavior changes.

There's a lot of ignorance and fear about autism. The stigma of autism is tremendous. No child wants to be labeled, and no parent wants their child to face isolation, shame, or struggle. Even high functioning autistic children face judgment at diagnosis, at school, and in social circles. This book shines a light on these misconceptions, and offers a way forward for parents, doctors and teachers to make a difference for children on the spectrum.

The stigma doesn't only affect the child. People often blame the parents because their child can't learn or focus, or may not be able to do tasks that other kids can do. Because mothers often bear the burden of managing their child's health, education, and discipline, they are often accused of bad parenting. Now that we know autism can be treated medically, these prejudices are outdated.

A diagnosis of autism is officially about communication and social skill deficits, but true autism awareness begins when we understand the world the way our friends on the spectrum do, and learn to understand the many reasons behind those deficits. There are many remedies to correct them. We can help our children overcome their overwhelming experiences and focus, learn and grow. Their experience is overwhelming because the world feels too loud, too crowded, too itchy, or too painful. The challenge is that remedies need to be custom fit to each child. Each child has individual needs and circumstances.

What we see as behavioral problems may have medical solutions. Autistic children, like all children, communicate through their behavior. Sometimes people don't understand what we can learn by paying attention to our children, who are showing us that they are in pain, even though they don't look sick. Friends and family may mean well, but their comments do not translate that way. "Oh, he doesn't look autistic." Or, "For an autistic kid, he's doing great," are not as positive as they could be. New research is opening our understanding about the medical problems behind autism, but the science is far from complete, and often complicated.

Parents go to the doctor and say "Johnny scratches his arms all day, runs around and won't eat." The doctor does not give the parent a cream for the itching or something to stop the diarrhea. If the parent suggests these things they are called a helicopter parent. The child is labeled as noncompliant, a picky eater or his scratching as an obsessive behavior. It should be common sense to resolve the medical issues first.

Our assumptions about children on the spectrum are often false. Parents often hear stories from experts that convince them their kids will never be able to accomplish anything. Our kids prove them wrong every day, not because they "grew out of it," or because autism went away on its own. Our hard work and love makes a difference for our kids. Every time our kids on the spectrum do something an expert said could not be done, we need to celebrate it together as a community.

I know from experience the value of clear information, community connections, and effective teams to support our kids. I'm the mother of two recovering children, both significantly improved because we dealt with the medical problems associated with their autistic symptoms. I have been researching autism for their recovery for ten years. My experience comes not just from my own identical twins, but from my work in our community as well. I've coached and supported many children with special needs, all with their own unique challenges. I also supported autistic adults in the 1980s, and I can only wish I knew then what I know now because I look back and see the same medical problems for the autism community. Out of respect for families reluctant to face stigma, including my own, every story in this book is true, but presented as a composite of people I've coached, interviewed, or supported.

I see many common challenges facing all people on the spectrum. Schools and group homes are not aware that medical and behavioral interventions are not mutually exclusive. Medical symptoms are connected to behaviors we consider to be autistic. We need to address both behavioral and medical issues, with all the experts on our team talking together. Without this collaboration, recovery can be slow or stalled.

Parents are the people who understand their children the best. Each person on the spectrum needs an alert parent to bridge the gap between all those experts to make certain that the goals are met. Parents are the liaison between different groups to be sure that everyone communicates well in the best interest of the child.

We really do know our children best and we should always have informed consent in medical care. Professionals sometimes disagree, even with each other, labeling the parents as helicopter parents for asking questions or calling them free range parents for not asking enough, instead of validating their concerns and honoring their questions. But there are ways to fight this prejudice, and to support our children and our families.

I've designed this book to help busy parents who must constantly watch their child, and who says, "I don't have time to read all the studies!" This book will help parents explain their children to the world, and help autistic children explain themselves when they are in pain. Like all children, they need to be taken seriously when they show pain symptoms, which should not be not dismissed by the doctors as "just autism" behavior. When a parent knows their child is in pain, the doctor should address that pain as they would with any other patient.

My goal is to share my expertise and research to reduce the stigma and confusion that can make a hard situation more challenging. Parents can use this book as a resource to advocate for their child with professionals, sharing it with people on their team who need a readable guide to understand the complexity of autism, as well as symptoms specific to their child. For the therapist or teacher, this book helps explain why our kids are medically sick, not just behaviorally challenged. For physicians, this book will help connect medical and behavioral issues as well as understanding how sickness affects how autistic kids think, learn or function.

If Only I Had Known....

My life has come full circle in the lessons I've learned about autism and toxicity. The medical issues of my children's autism symptoms came from the same root of chronic fatigue and debilitating pain in me. These medical issues run in families even when the autism does not. My medical history was an indication that that I could not naturally detoxify myself and neither could my children. If I had known then what I know now, I might have lessened their autism or even prevented it.

The stories in this book explore real experiences of overwhelming pain resulting from poor immune system function, gut and brain disconnection, toxicity, vaccines, environmental problems, and genetics, as well as viruses and Lyme disease. Parents who understand how to look for these indicators may decrease the chances of having a child on the spectrum and improve the health and wellbeing of the whole family.

Doctors were at first doubtful about the sources of my pain, but tests, research and treatment led to significant relief. They could have figured it out if they had put in the time and research, but I had to do it myself, and then find a doctor who would help me heal. My headaches were really the mercury from my teeth in my jaw. My Irritable Bowel Syndrome was gluten intolerance, allergies and Candida. My chronic fatigue was Lyme Disease.

As I researched autism, I decided to have the same doctor I found for my children examine me, to relieve my symptoms of pain and anguish and finally get a proper diagnosis and treatment. I know what this pain is that our children experience, because I lived with it longer than anyone should. My doctor told me that if I had not gone to him, I would have had cancer, because my immunity was so low, my pain was high, and my toxicity was off the chart. The research I am presenting saved my life and helped my children. Now they can speak when experts said they would not ever have a real conversation.

Sometimes doctors will curb the behaviors or lower the stress levels with medications. This kind of treatment may or may not work. At its worst, it has bad side effects. It may take many years of different medications to find the one that works, and in the meantime, the ones that do not work can make behavior worse for a limited time, or cause a new behavioral symptom. Sometimes, when the system works at its best, the child is calmer but still in pain.

I began my coaching and extended my research by joining Defeat Autism Now conferences (DAN). Founded by the late Bernie Rimland, a microbiologist with an adult child on the spectrum, these conferences supported a community to explore a new idea, that autism is not just genetic or behavioral, and it has no connection to parents who were too cold to their children, known as refrigerator mothers. He was one of the first scientists who acknowledged the complexity of autism, because he was also a parent with an affected child. With autism increasing in our populations, parents who are also doctors are now becoming experts and guides.

I followed the communities that developed after DAN, tracking new research so I could be a resource for other parents. These doctors left DAN and to form a new group called Medical Academy of Pediatric Special Needs (MAPS).

After the DAN conferences ended I attended other conferences to talk to the experts, including the National Vaccine Information Center and Autism One. In these communities, I met Dr. Andrew Wakefield, Dr. Joe Mercola, Jenny McCarthy, Dr. Brian Hooker PhD, and Dr. Stephanie Seneff, Ph.D., whose work has shaped a new way to understand autism and its treatments.

Learning from these doctors and scientists made me realize that my professional background was as useful as my experience with my own children on the spectrum. I worked in the Freedom of Information office, and as a contractor at Astra Merck pharmaceutical company. I learned how the system works, and how the drug approval process works to submit drugs to the FDA.

I shared my research through many networks with other parents, using social media and support groups. As I was finishing my research, I gathered more stories for this book through my radio show, Kitchen Sink Autism: Everything but the Kitchen Sink about autism, featured on Blog Talk Radio from 2010-2012. I wanted to ground my research in first hand experiences because not all autism is the same. I learned that not all autism is associated with vaccines, and not all vaccine injuries are about autism. I wanted to know everything about every symptom, every treatment, or therapy whether or not my kids needed them. Through my research, I found the stories of Lisa Mark Smith, Linda Weinmaster, and Virginia Young, important stories shared in this book.

Over the years, I have introduced parents with kids with similar issues, and helped them find doctors and other team members. I helped facilitate support through Talk About Curing Autism Now. I also was a "rescue angel" at Generation Rescue, facilitating mentoring connections between new and experienced parents to identify local services. My coaching work now involves mentoring parents about possible treatments and helping build working relationships with professionals. My doctor referred patients to me because they did not see treatments as necessary and did not start because they were expensive. I do not diagnose or treat the kids but I help translate behavioral problems to support a child's medical needs. I sometimes call a school or a therapist to support parents and children. This book includes much of the information I give to parents to explain to the school how and why the child was getting treatments from their doctor.

The toughest part of this journey is getting started and knowing where to begin. Many parents try to study autism, but without a system or a guide, they become confused as to how to begin. In my research and coaching, I've found that all autism families have at least one of these categories: Lyme, toxicity, vaccines, and the gut/brain/immunity connection. In this book, I explore each of these issues, with stories of children with these issues to help parents sort out which problem applies to their family.

How can parents use this book?

This is the book I wish I had when my kids were first diagnosed. It includes detailed information often shared by coaches and mentors to get started as quickly as possible. It will help you learn what is important for your child and what is not.

Although professionals can use the information here, this book is primarily for parents with children on the spectrum. Parents are constantly explaining their autistic child's behavior, medications, side effects, supplements, special diets, allergies and other problems to everyone who encounters that child. This book helps parents communicate with their children, and with their treatment and education teams by identifying the connections between medical conditions and behavior.

These behaviors are clues to what the child is experiencing and feeling, a form of communication if we are aware of it. Therapists and teachers tell us how to deal with disruptive autistic behaviors in school settings, but they may not know the medical reasons. Medical doctors tell us what is physically wrong, but may not help us handle the behaviors. This book will help you interpret and respond to your child better, not just by collecting important information, but also by learning to interpret what they are trying to tell you, without words.

Kids on the spectrum often have some combination of system damage that can be diagnosed and treated. These include gut, immune, brain, toxicity or vaccine damage, Lyme disease or some combination. Most of them have issues with foods that can make behavior worse, including MSG or GMOs, and other toxins in the Standard American Diet. (SAD). These influences affect your child's health and behavior. This book will help you to be able to identify the ones that affect your child, and find tools to help them feel better.

As you read this book, think about what you would do if you had a deficit in social and communication skills and you were in tremendous pain and could not tell anyone. What things do you do to show the world your pain? Imagine it from their point of view: if you had an itch you'd scratch it. If you had diarrhea you would run to find a bathroom even if you did not know where the bathroom was. If you knew that food caused pain, you wouldn't eat.

A lot of people still expect us to give up, accepting the diagnosis as an automatic disability. As you'll find in this book, even if we can't help our children on the spectrum overcome every challenge, we can help them feel more comfortable so they can be more successful and happy.

Your child may be communicating discomfort, or pain, or stress by his behaviors. Some places simply want to medicate for these behaviors, which may calm the child temporarily, but if the parent or teacher does not understand what the child is trying to tell them, the behaviors will not stop. My ideal world would be one where the teachers and therapists understand children's medical needs, and know that children may need multiple medications, vitamins or supplements, or even special diets. We shouldn't have to explain what we know is necessary again and again.

By helping you identify the underlying medical problems that complicate your child's world, this book will help you prepare you to handle any necessary treatment your doctor provides. It will also help you avoid exchanging treatments with your friends, because you will understand your child's system so well you won't waste time treating a problem your child doesn't have.

Experienced parents as well as parents of newly diagnosed children can use this book to increase autism awareness, and as a tool to erase the stigma of autism that shadows your family. They can share it with family, friends and neighbors, and offer it as evidence at their child's IEP meetings. They can even leave a copy at the doctor's office, for the doctor or other new parents.

Of course, I am not specifically diagnosing your child. This is a learning tool to simplify the process of your investigation of your child's experience, identify his health challenges and lessen pain so that the child is ready to learn. I have simplified as much as possible in the appendix to explain medical diagnoses that can create troublesome behaviors, what a healthy bowel movement looks like, terminology of services in school, and how his immunity, gut, and toxicity are all connected. I have also included a guide to the autism diets and how to identify problematic foods. The stories help explain how behaviors can be expressions of pain and what she may be trying to tell you.

Autism is a marathon, not a sprint. It takes a long time to help our kids. Of course, the earlier you begin the better, but it's never too late. True autism awareness begins with awareness of the pain and identifying what the child is trying to tell you, step by step. My hope is that it will also be part of changing the way the world sees our kids and us as parents, ultimately erasing the autism stigma, one family at a time.

"One person can make a difference, and everyone should try."
-JFK

Part 1: The Gut, The Brain and the Immune System

David: The Poop Decorator

David had skinny little arms and legs and big protruding belly as if he had swallowed a beach ball. Four years old, he was still wearing a pull up diaper. He looked like a typical child except for the smell of excrement that seemed to linger wherever he went. David could not tell his mother when he needed to "go" with words, but sometimes his behavior gave her some hints. He looked at her silently, as if he was screaming with his eyes, Sometimes, he yelled and shrieked, but it wasn't always clear to her that what was triggering his behavior.

The walls, the floor, and the sink was decorated in David's poop. He didn't like it on his finger but it hurt him to poop so he often used his finger to get it out. He wiped the poop anywhere within reach, the floor, the toilet paper, the sink, or the clean towel his mom used for company.

His mother didn't want to invite anyone over because the bathroom was decorated with poop stains and David was always hiding behind a chair squatting in the corner and screaming. He screamed so loudly when he was constipated that the neighbors called the police.

When he had to go to the bathroom it was sudden and he would get up from where ever he was and run. But sometimes he could not get his pants down fast enough to reach the toilet. He was embarrassed about this, so he hid behind a chair in a squat, pooping where no one could see. He didn't like the feel of the poop on his bare skin so sometimes he took his clothes off and walked around without pants, leaving his dirty clothes on the floor for his mother to find later.

David walked around clenching his behind and walking on his tiptoes, trying very hard not to soil himself and to do his best to be discreet and hide it when he did. He was in a constant panic. His mother told him hundreds of times how to use the toilet and where to go. She carried around raisins to reward him when he was successful but he still couldn't make it to the bathroom.

David's mom knew where every bathroom was in every store and whenever she took him somewhere, she always took him there first thing. She carried a backpack with her everywhere she went with a few changes of clothes for David, because she never knew when she would need them. She could shop for anything in ten minutes, which is all the time they had before he had to poop again.

Sometimes his poop was slimy diarrhea. Sometimes it looked like hard little rabbit pellets. When he was constipated, he didn't poop for a week, then clogged the toilet to the point that it would not flush. Doctors said that his constipation and diarrhea were just part of autism and gave him a stool softener called Miralax, which he took for years.

David and his mother did not know that his diet greatly influenced whether that day's symptom was diarrhea or constipation. He and his mother both craved the same foods even though they were causing digestive problems for both. He only would eat three or four things and she did not have the energy to cook, so she gave him those foods anyway. He was a picky eater, so she gave him what he liked to make sure he ate enough.

His favorite foods were McDonald's chicken nuggets and Lays potato chips, and she occasionally rewarded him (and herself!) with pizza. He also liked the weekends, when his mom would cook eggs. He was usually constipated during the week, and had diarrhea on the weekends.

David had numerous inflammation problems, viruses and food allergies. His mother sent him to a gastroenterologist who gave him a test for food allergies. He was allergic to eggs, soy, wheat and milk and numerous other minor allergens. He needed a periodic clean out of his bowels to prevent the constipation, even after he completely changed what he ate. His gut had a lot of healing left to do and it would be a long road to reduce the inflammation that made everyone's life miserable.

His doctor had to look inside his intestines to see why food was such a problem. The doctor had him swallow a pill that had a camera in (a pill cam) to look at what was wrong with this gut, and found evidence of the measles virus in his intestines. The doctor said his intestinal wall looked like raw hamburger, gooey and not pink and smooth at all. David started taking antivirals for the viruses and antifungals for the yeast.

Still, the inflammation was so bad it was painful for David to eat anything. For a time, he was drinking his vegetables, because his mother would juice some carrots, and apple and some cucumber, and he would drink that with a little bit of salt and pepper. She had to squirt it in his mouth, a teaspoon at a time. She made him smoothies with extra nutrition, and supplements mixed in, and others mixed into his applesauce. This was the first time he had really eaten fruits and vegetables. He drank smoothies with coconut milk, and strawberries with some stevia and ice. He loved that, even when it had some extra vitamins for his gut.

The supplements he took were liquid or powder form, so the only way he would eat them, was to be mixed with fruit. He could continue to eat the fruit for the time being because that's the only way he would eat his vegetables.

The allergy test and liquid/supplement diet was a first step to a modified diet, eliminating processed foods. It was not just his mother that had a learning curve, but David as well. They began a step-by-step process to learn that gluten and casein were the proteins in wheat and milk, which created a whole new David when he would indulge. He was sweet and gave her a hug when he complied, and he was constipated, nauseous and angry when he did not. Sometimes his behavior became worse because she did not realize she had given him gluten foods by mistake.

It took a few months of trial and error to find foods that fit his healthiest diet *and* that he would eat. This was a constant challenge. He could smell cheese and bread where ever it was, and begged for them like a starving dog. Sometimes, she could not resist, and gave him the foods, but would regret the change in behavior when she did. She had to learn the hard way not to keep cheese in the house, yet still find something that satisfied that creamy texture that he craved.

When she had a full seven-day menu that was completely gluten and casein free including juicing his vegetables and smoothies for dessert, she gave him the same foods over and over. He was now considered completely Gluten Fee Casein Free, which helped him considerably. After doing this diet for six months, David's behavior was calmer. He was no longer screaming, or smearing his poop all over the place.

She was now beginning to potty train him and he complied because it was so much easier for him. Now his poop was smooth like a snake, as it should be. David was still having occasional accidents but this was directly related to whether he complied with the diet. If he could stay away from the wrong foods, he was happier. As if letting air out of a balloon; his stomach shrank as the antifungals worked. He did not crave carbohydrates as often as he had before. If he cheated and ate a cracker, his mother had to start over, give him some activated charcoal, to get the cracker out of his system and time to work its way out of his body. That one cracker started the cravings all over again, as if he were an alcoholic having a sip of champagne.

After the medical intervention, David continued therapy to teach him what things are called, and used pictures to tell her what he wants. He was in a calmer, more relaxed space and eager to learn more. The therapy helped to ease frustrations because he was no longer learning new skills with such pain. (The first word he learned was "cheese!")

The best news was that the diarrhea and constipation were gone, and David did not need the pull-ups or changes of clothes. He no longer decorated his house with poop. He still had some distance to go with language learning, but if he had his iPad and could tell his mom what he wanted, he was more expressive. David was far from recovered from autism, but he was toilet trained -- mostly.

Tools for David and his Family

David's behavior of hiding behind furniture, poop smearing and his alternating diarrhea and constipation are all symptoms of gut problems. If the child has obvious gut problems, changing diet is the simplest thing to try. Common diets are discussed in Part 5 of this book. Not every child with autism has gut problems, but improving the gut will improve behaviors if the behaviors are indications of stomach pain.

David was taking off his dirty clothes because he did not like the feel of messing his pants. His parents can use that as motivation such as letting him wear his favorite clothes if he can keep them on and clean. If David really likes Spiderman, his parents could buy him Spiderman pajamas, but only let him wear them if he can keep them dry.

Miralax is for short-term use only.[1] The FDA has explained that it can cause neuropsychiatric events in users. A stool analysis can help to understand why he has problems with his gastrointestinal tract. Read about dietary changes and remedies to find out alternatives to Miralax. He may need to periodic clean outs to make sure he had normal bowel movements.

Parents can keep a diary to monitor his eating to determine what foods may be causing pain, diarrhea or constipation as well as negative behaviors. The fact that he has diarrhea on the weekends means they need to look at everything he eats at that time. If his behavior or his bowels change when he eats McDonald's, he may need to avoid it to see if the behavior or physical pains are reduced. His mother needed to decide whether the trip to McDonald's was worth dealing with the behavior that came with it. The food diary and the behavior charts work together, because he is calmer if he improves his diet, and some behaviors relate to food reactions

Some kids won't eat because the new food is a change in routine. If he will only eat McDonald's, she can give him homemade chicken nuggets in a McDonalds bag. She could sprinkle potato chip crumbs on a new food like green beans and make sure David sees her do it. He may eat a few green beans too.
*Some kids need strict GFCF compliance and this strategy is not recommended for kids with full celiac.
Using the Poop Chart in Appendix A, she will need to monitor his poop. How many a day? What it looks like? Is it painful? Then get a Comprehensive Stool Analysis from Great Plains Labs to determine bacteria, yeast, allergies and parasites. His poop should look smooth like a snake just like Type 4 in Appendix A of the Bristol Stool Chart.
David's protruding belly is a sign of yeast overgrowth. Yeasty kids crave carbohydrates and sugar. Since macaroni and cheese, and pizza are his favorite foods, David's parents should consider the possibility of an addiction to sugar, influenced by yeast in the gut, and another addiction to the gluten and casein. Some kids can feel a high from these foods. Parents may find that this runs in families and the whole family may have yeast problems, and have food addictions.

Why Is the Gut Important in Autism?

Medical professionals have been saying for years that autism is generally a brain disorder. Parents with kids on the spectrum see a lot of gut dysfunction and wonder if autism problems are associated with the gut. The brain, the gut, and the immune system are intimately connected. We cannot look at one without looking at all three.

Emerging science demonstrates that the problems begin by an imbalance between these three systems can no longer be dismissed as "just autism." We know that healing the gut will also heal the brain and vice versa.

The brain and the gut have much in common. Each has vital nerve systems and key connections with immune function. Chemical imbalances of serotonin and dopamine, once only thought to be in the brain, are also reflected in the gut.

Doctors treating mental health should also consider what happens to the gut when they correct this chemical imbalance with drugs. Serotonin is a chemical that regulates bowel function, mood, blood clotting, stomach health, bone density and sexual function. It is produced in our intestines.[2] Toxoplasma Gondii is a parasite usually found in the gut can increase dopamine.[3] Too many doctors treat chemical imbalances of brain disorders without considering that their patients may become imbalanced because of the gut consequences.

The healthy bacteria found in the gut are also important because it is your protector to keep toxicity out of the body. Gut bacteria are a "tuning fork of the immune system." The gut provides a natural barrier to environmental toxins, and we eliminate those toxins naturally when we throw up. If the gut is not functioning properly, 'gut dysbiosis' results, creating an abnormal amount of gut flora and digestive/immune/behavior problems.[4] Thus, we may be eating our vegetables, but are unable to absorb their nutritional value and some foods pass through the digestive system whole and we can see their remnants in the poop. Your child may not necessarily get the vitamins needed within the good food you provide.

Your gut lining is a protector to keep out unwanted food particles or anything that causes the gut to be damaged. Intestinal permeability or leaky gut means that the molecules pass through the gut lining that should not.[5] Seventy percent of our immune system is found in the gut.[6] If we bypass this built-in immunity, our body can't fight back properly.

The brain and the gut are also connected because our gut has its own set of nerves, "the second brain," per Michael Gershon. "The Enteric Nervous System contains 100 million neurons, more than the spinal cord or peripheral nervous system."[7]

The brain also has immune function. "The brain is like every other tissue connected to the peripheral immune system through meningeal lymphatic vessels," said Jonathan Kipnis, a professor at the University of Virginia in the Department of Neuroscience. "They'll have to rewrite the textbooks,"[8] said Kevin Lee, who chairs the department, when Dr. Kipnis shared the results with him.

The American Academy of Pediatrics acknowledges that the ASD population has gastrointestinal issues such as abdominal pain and constipation including abdominal pain, diarrhea, constipation, and unusually high rate of GI disorders.[9, 10] There is a strong connection between Irritable Bowel Syndrome and depression and anxiety. Specialists should know how these conditions affect one another,[11] but only specialize in one part of the body and miss these connections.

The gut becomes damaged in the foods we eat and the chemicals and toxins we encounter. Inflammation, viruses, MSG, GMOs, reactions to foods, vaccines, allergies, parasites, lack of nutrients, toxins, antibiotics, bottle feeding, prescription medications, birth control pills, processed foods carbohydrates all influence the gut flora.[12] Sometimes parents and doctors will excuse an unhealthy gut as "just autism." As I interviewed parents, they said things like, "Johnny pooped once a month. That was normal for him. Then his poop was the size of a softball and it clogged the toilet." Another said, "Oh, don't worry, he poops by the gallon. It gushes out of him." These are extreme versions of constipation and diarrhea and they are not normal bowel movements even if they are what your child has always done.

The way your child poops, how often, its consistency, uniformity, size and color has direct correlation with his health, his mood, and his symptoms of autism. A healthy gut should have two bowel movements a day. Overall, good gut health results in feeling well after eating, sleeping soundly, having energy throughout the day, experiencing a steady mood, and enjoying a balanced diet without food cravings[13].

The Most Frequent Complaints of Those on the Spectrum

- Chronic diarrhea
- Gas
- Abdominal discomfort
- Distension
- Mal-absorption[14]

Gastrointestinal inflammation may make ASD symptoms worse. Dietary interventions can ease GI inflammation in at least some children.[15] Sometimes, when whole families shift their dietary behaviors, everyone's health is improved, not just the health of children on the spectrum, because these gut issues may be problems for several people in the family. Special diets can help correct them.

Parent and child may need to stop eating gluten for different reasons. The mother might have chronic fatigue and irritable bowel syndrome, and the child has autism, but both have a problem eating gluten, and both benefit from a GFCF (Gluten Free/Casein Free) diet in different ways. Sometimes parents may not even realize their diet is the problem, until they have a child on the spectrum who cannot eat certain foods. The health of the whole family improves because they wanted to help their son, and changed everyone's food plan.

It's important to remember that behaviors are associated with multiple medical problems; so, supporting gut health may not relieve all a child's autistic symptoms. However, I've seen significant shifts in some families and my own children. Even when behaviors don't disappear (and sometimes they do!), reducing pain, shortening the time it takes for a child to recover, and toning down the behaviors themselves can make a big difference for both a child and family.

Specific Behavioral Symptoms of an Unhealthy Gut

"Stooping" or pushing on the stomach

Some children may lean over furniture or lie with their stomachs over a swing, or push in their stomach. This pressure-based self-treatment makes their stomachs feel better. It's a clear sign of gut problems. If this self-treatment doesn't work, a child may scream to express the pain and the strong emotions of frustration. Stimming, flapping hands, clicking fingers or other repeated self-stimulation is another way autistic kids will release energy or try to cope with feeling overwhelmed. Pay attention to these self-soothing behaviors to get a clue to the source of the pain. Sometimes kids can be excited and happy as well, still feeling overwhelmed, so kids will stim for different reasons.

Poop smearing

Chronically constipated children endure a great deal of pain and embarrassment. It might be hard to eliminate small, hard, poop. A natural solution is to pull it out them, with a finger. Because many children on the autism spectrum are already sensitive to textures, smells and dirt, the mess will be triggering. They will wipe it off anywhere they can: on a chair, the table the wall or the floor, anything to get it off their hands. Healing the gut makes this behavior less likely.

Toilet readiness

A child with autism may not be able to tell you that he must go to the bathroom, but his nonverbal signs are the same as any toddler ready to begin toilet training. Your child may be 26 but still show the same nonverbal signs, like grunting, squatting or stripping off his clothes when it's time to go.[16] Helping him maintain a healthy gut will make toilet training easier for both of you.

Eating Dirt and Sand

When a child eats dirt or sand or something that is a non-food item, it's known as PICA. Kids are looking for something that's missing in their diet like zinc or iron.[17] Providing the child with supplements and improving gut health allows them to absorb the zinc will relieve this sometimes-disturbing symptom.

What Gets in the Way?

Sugar and Carbohydrates

Yeast overgrowth, or Candida, behaviors are worsened by excess consumption of sugar and carbs. Candida can create physical symptoms like ulcers and colitis, and behavioral symptoms.[18] Excess yeast is linked to a whole range of symptoms from fatigue and depression to hyperactivity and anger.[19] *Talk about Curing Autism Now* has a full list of symptoms. I have listed these in Appendix

B.[20] There is a useful test called a comprehensive stool analysis to test for yeast by Great Plains Laboratories.[21]

Sugar can lower immune function and an excess of sugar feeds the Candida causing yeast infections.[22] When the immune system is not functioning, the body does not produce antibodies.[23] The immune system is less efficient with an excess of sugar.

The next story is about Joey who liked to climb things and was quite hyperactive. He is an example of a child addicted to sugar and carbohydrates, and might benefit from one of the diets mentioned in this book. His story explains how a child's behaviors reflect sugar and carbohydrate addictions and why the GFCF diet and Candida diet may offer him some benefit.

Joey: The Climber

Joey was six years old, short for his age and bone thin. He was so skinny you could see his ribs and the bones in his arms and legs. His stomach, however looked like a big beach ball and it made gurgling noises at the most inappropriate times. He had red chapped lips and he licked them as if they were always covered in candy. He squirmed in his chair, using the chair to scratch his behind. Joey's sleeves always had holes because he chewed on the edge of his sleeves. He liked to poke his thumb through the holes, and sometimes sucked on his fingers.

Joey never slept more than two hours in a row. He liked to wake up at two a.m. and laugh. For some reason the lights that reflected off the ceiling seem to have little colors and shapes that were entertaining to him as if they were alive. He would watch them and point at them for his mom, Kathy, to see but she had no idea what he was pointing to and just once wanted to sleep all the way through the night. Joey would flap his hands, excitedly as he watched the colors reflect from the hallway light that he insisted had to be on at all times. He didn't have to speak to tell her he wanted the lights on. If she turned them off, he turned them back on and the battle kept going until she was frustrated and left them on. He had to have the door open at just the right angle, and wear his favorite blue socks at night.

Joey never seemed to have his feet on the ground. He climbed the jungle gym, the couch, the dining room table, or the bookshelf. He was like a little monkey climbing from one piece of furniture to another as if the floor was made of lava. Kathy knew never to put cookies up on a high shelf because that is the first place he would look, and it only motivated him to climb where it was not safe.

Joey ate food as if it were a drug he needed, especially any kind of cookies or bread, or other foods with sugar or gluten. He would inhale the aroma and then eat the treat in one gulp, barely chewing. Kathy couldn't keep milk, cheese, cookies, bread, cereal or cake in the house because it was like Joey had a super nose and seemed to smell where she hid his favorites, especially cookies. She frequently would find the empty cookie container soon after she had restocked the shelf.

Joey's cravings for cookies were as strong as an addict's hunger for cocaine. His behavior changed as if he were high when he ate cookies. His teacher gave him cookies for rewards when he was calm at school, but then he would try to grab the whole box and steal them from other children. For a while the sugar explosion in his gut gave him a huge burst of energy, and away he went like a little monkey climbing on the furniture.

After he came down, his eyes were glassy with big blue streaks under them and he seemed to be somewhere else. He would crash about an hour after his snack and slump down, sitting on the couch and staring into empty space. Kathy called it a "cookie coma." He would become so exhausted and burnt out that his memory was the first thing to go.

Depending on what he ate and how much, he had trouble at school with learning and behavior. When he was high on sugar, the radio was louder to him, the coffee maker buzzed and people talking to him felt like they were shouting, so he would shout back as if he were next to the speakers at a rock concert.

Kathy begrudgingly did her best to take care of him but the truth was she wasn't well herself. When she stood up too quickly, she would see blackness in the lower half of her vision, and she would sit down until her head was clear again. When she stood up, her whole body ached especially the back of her legs. She had to watch Joey even when she felt sick, and was burnt out and exhausted.

Even though she suspected that the cookies were a real problem, Kathy couldn't stop buying them because she craved them as intensely as he did, although she would never admit that to anyone. She was overweight but just never felt full and even though she already felt sick, she kept eating anyway, as if she was punishing herself. Her stomach was so bloated she looked pregnant even though she wasn't.

Kathy's hips were often painful and she frequently had cramps in the middle of the night so she would toss and turn to feel comfortable. When she woke up, in pain, she had to think about where to go and what to do, down to small details because movement was painful. Still, she had certain things she thought had to be done and worked herself beyond exhaustion.

Since she was not sleeping very soundly, she awoke easily with Joey. She frequently would go to his room to try to comfort him. She was not even sure if she could sleep much anyway, because her stomach pains kept her awake.

If anyone asked, Kathy always had the appearance that everything was great, because her house was very clean and her lawn was well manicured. She cleaned the house at night when she couldn't sleep. She sometimes woke up at midnight exhausted but wide-awake. Sometimes she would pull up a chair to wash dishes because she could not stand up very long but also could not sleep. She worked until she couldn't move and every bone and muscle and joint in her body ached, but kept going even at three in the morning like a zombie. She was awake, but half asleep, pushing through her pain because movement made her feel better. Occasionally, exhaustion made her sit back down, but she would get up again quickly, because she was so uncomfortable.

When it was bedtime for Joey he was just like his mother. He worked hard at the things that he thought were important. However, his idea of important was different than hers. He tried hard to show her the lights on the ceiling and how to climb bookshelves. He would climb everything until he just could not get moving and would sit and rub his sore achy feet. Sometimes the two of them sat and rubbed each other's feet because it felt so good to not be standing up. Joey would crash hard and sleep all day and all night and then not sleep again for weeks.

Both Joey and his mother needed to begin a Paleo diet to eliminate sugar and carbohydrates to feel better. Their addictions were overwhelming as they would often start and stop over and over, learning as they struggled. He needed a new reward at school so that he could thrive and pay attention. He also needed to take probiotics with a strong antifungal treatment to eliminate the yeast in his gut. His doctor recommended a test called a stool analysis to find out what was happening in his gut.

This would become an ongoing struggle for this family and I cannot say that they completely overcame sugar and gluten addiction. His behaviors continued to go away and then come back again, depending on his diet that day.

Sugar imbalance is very difficult to overcome but the trick is to realize the consequences of eating the wrong foods, and working with the behaviors that need to be corrected. Some people can go without sugar for a while and then eat it in moderation, but some can't. It depends how the body heals and levels of allergies. It depends on the child.

Tools for Joey's Family

Joey has certain behaviors to indicate food addictions. He goes into a food "coma," getting glassy-eyed, he became hyper and then crashed when the sugar high wore off. A specialized diet (see suggestions for David) can make a big difference.

Some of Joey's signs of yeast were that he climbed furniture, didn't sleep, laughed for no reason, and chewed on his sleeves.

He has physical signs with the behavioral signs such as under eye circles, glassy eyed, big round belly, and not sleeping well.

Kathy may need to find another venue where climbing is appropriate such as a park or a jungle gym or rock climbing if it is age appropriate.

If she cannot eliminate sugar completely she can taper it down. Stevia and Xylitol can be good substitutes for sugar. He can also have lemons and limes because they make the body more alkaline and lessen sugar cravings. She can make Paleo versions of lemon custard or key lime pie using xylitol to help with the sugar cravings but still comply with the diet.

Some suggestions to improve sleep include going to bed at the same time and waking up at the same time every day, turning off all electronic devices an hour before bed, spending time at the end of the day relaxing even if you are not tired, and not to eat anything that might upset the stomach before bed.

Remedies for a good healthy sleep include taking a warm bath with a cup of Epsom salt, a drop of lavender essential oil, and a tablespoon of baking soda. The Epsom salt has magnesium to be absorbed through the skin, the lavender will help put the body in a state of relaxation, and the baking soda helps the body to be more alkaline.

Kathy can also check with the doctor to find out if there are any medical reasons why Joey isn't sleeping.

Other Food Issues

Genetically Modified Foods (GMOs)

Recent studies indicate that GMOs deplete amino acids like tryptophan, damage DNA, and disrupt gut bacteria, lowering the effectiveness of the immune system. Dr. Stephanie Seneff from MIT reports that glyphosate, an ingredient in Round Up and Round Up ready foods is associated with autism as well as heart disease, obesity, diabetes, gastrointestinal disorders, infertility, and cancer. The shikimate pathway that synthesizes essential amino acids present in gut bacteria is blocked from consumption of glyphosate. Organic foods do not contain glyphosate. [24] Appendix C lists the foods listed known as the dirty dozen, foods you should always eat organic because they are almost always GMO.

Monosodium Glutamate (MSG)

MSG is a flavor enhancer that also acts as a neurotoxin, overexciting the neurons so they die. MSG makes mediocre food taste good, and you will keep eating when you are full. Some of the behaviors resulted by MSG are migraines, binge eating, screaming because of pain, no eye contact, insomnia, seizures, anger and depression. [25]

Ironically, many of the drugs prescribed to cure the diseases and disorders mentioned above are glutamate blockers. The FDA has declared MSG to be safe, but at the same time, has approved glutamate blockers. As informed consumers, we should not be paying for MSG and then paying for a drug to remove it. [26]

Children on the spectrum should avoid any further damage and behavioral complications by avoiding MSG. It is still generally considered safe by the FDA.[27]

MSG is hidden in most everyday foods. It is in just about every processed food and in vaccines. You may not know you are eating it because it has many names. Appendix D is a list of ingredients that contain MSG. Appendix E lists the foods that sometimes contain MSG. Sometimes there are many of these in the same food which might give the illusion that there is less MSG except that it is listed many times in the same food if you know what to look for. Additionally, the behaviors of MSG are difficult to spot because how much MSG is in each food is not labeled correctly and since the effect tis cumulative, one cannot tell how much they are consuming. These behaviors are things like depression, mood swings and lethargy as well as physical symptoms of migraines, rapid heartbeat, and joint pain.[28]

Not Absorbing Nutrients

Parents often work hard to make sure their kids are eating healthy foods, so they don't understand why they would need extra vitamins or supplements. Many of our kids have intestinal permeability which allow toxicity to enter the blood. This can result in undigested food to travel through the gastrointestinal tract, limiting absorption of nutrients and vitamins along with it. You can identify this problem by examining your child's poop. If you can tell what the child ate and see remnants of food in their poop, then they're not absorbing the nutrients they need.[29]

In a study of juvenile delinquents, violence and serious antisocial behavior were cut almost in half after implementing nutrient-dense diets.[30] Another study showed antisocial behavior in prisons, including violence, is reduced by adding vitamins, minerals and essential fatty acids. The implications are clear for those eating poor diets in the community.[31]

Here are some common vitamins that our children may lack:

Zinc or Iron	PICA or eating non-food items reflects a lack of iron or zinc in the diet. Children with PICA desire textures in their mouth.[32]
Vitamin D	Known as "the sunshine vitamin" because we get vitamin D naturally from the sun. Rickets, a disease from the lack of Vitamin D can cause brittle bones or bones that break easily.[33] Parents of children with healing Rickets are sometimes accused of child abuse, because that is what the body looks like.[34]
Vitamin C	Barlow's disease or scurvy manifests as broken bones, bruising, and sores that do not heal. It can also look like the child was abused. Test for Vitamin C deficiency if that happens.[35]

Synergistic Effects

These factors create a cascading effect on the gut, the brain and the immune system. Most people have their own combination of factors. They build on each other and make symptoms worse. Low-grade encephalopathy is associated with exposure to nitric oxide, ammonia and glutamate in the central nervous system. Environmental factors can synergistically promote the encephalopathy of autism, which is also complicated by the herbicide glyphosate, aluminum, mercury, lead, nutritional deficiencies in thiamine and zinc, and yeast overgrowth due to excess dietary sugar. [36] Doctors are consistently finding new syndromes, chemicals and genes that are causing autism. If the problem is that people have genes that limit their ability to excrete chemicals properly, then environmental and food allergies or gluten intolerance can only make symptoms worse.

How Do We Make the Gut Healthy Again?

In simplistic terms, the best thing parents can do is to heal what's broken, remove what's causing harm, and replace what's missing. If the problem is inflammation or diarrhea we can relieve the pain or reduce inflammation with medications or supplements, so that the child can eat without pain. We figure out if there are any foods or anything in his environment making this situation worse. Do certain foods make him vomit, or have diarrhea or constipation? If the problem is allergies, we figure out what the child is allergic to, and remove that food from their diet. If there are metals like mercury or other toxins, removal of those not just from the environment but also from the body is the next step. If the child is malnourished or can't absorb certain vitamins or nutrients we offer supplements to give the child what she lacks. This sounds like common sense, but in the physical symptoms of an autistic child are sometimes not taken seriously.

Healing the gut is the first step in the child's ability to curb unwanted behaviors and further reduce injuries by avoiding toxicity, or excluding foods that a child cannot tolerate or digest completely. Both are an extensive learning curve, take time, and are expensive. Each child is unique.

Your child's toxicity, their gut problems, and their immune function are different from your friend's child.

I have included some natural ways to help the body heal, because much of this overlaps through all the whole book. If this is your main concern, you can skip to that part, but I would suggest you read through to understand the way symptoms and solutions overlap.

Part 2: How Does Lyme Disease Affect Behavior and Physical Health?

Pete: The Refuser

Peter was a happy, smart, twelve-year-old who was exceptional on the computer. He did not need anyone to teach him how to fix his computer, and he even installed a new operating system all by himself. He learned how to make his own music videos with his own green screen. He experimented with sound, lighting and backgrounds to do all kinds of interesting videos, without anyone teaching him or from taking classes. It was his natural talent.

Overnight, Pete's mood suddenly changed from happy to depressed. He was suddenly not physically or emotionally able to handle his life when he could easily cope before. He slept very little, waking up with head, neck and hip pain.

Pete refused to make videos or use the computer and spent his evenings crying instead because he felt so sick. His main symptoms were a mild headache, fever, chills and sleepiness. His doctor thought he had the beginnings of the flu, but the symptoms didn't pass. Pete began losing his short-term memory, and his mood changed to depression and anger, even escalating into violent outbursts. His fingers and hands hurt as if he had arthritis.

He failed tests that used to be easy for him. Pete's memory just was not what it used to be. He forgot facts and dates he had to remember for tests. He forgot details of his stories, people's names and faces, and he frequently got lost. He forgot his supplies to go from class to class. He forgot ingredients to make a chocolate cake, even though he had made this cake many times before.

Pete's inability to do even simple things caused him great aggravation. Anything in his environment that might have changed from the day before made him intensely angry. He would throw objects, even threatened to harm himself when he was stressed, or hit others or himself.

Mostly his anger expressed his own frustration. He would say, "I'm such an idiot," or "This is stupid," or "I knew the answer!" He ripped up or scribbled on the paper when he failed at tests because he forgot the answers. His teachers were at a loss to explain his behavior changes or why his grades continued to drop. Some didn't know he had been an A student the year before.

Pete's hands and wrists were swollen and painful. His knees cracked and he lost some flexibility. His hands were hurting so he refused to use a pen or pencil and he needed frequent breaks. He refused to play sports or any sort of activity in PE that involved a lot of movement. Soon, Pete would no longer participate at all in PE. Simply walking to class was hard, but running around the track was next to impossible. He would rather lie down on the floor and sleep because he was chronically exhausted. Sometimes, this is exactly what he did.

Pete had been to therapists, psychologists, and medical personnel who tried to figure out what was wrong with him. One psychologist prescribed anti-anxiety meds like Xanax and said it was all in his head. He had started physical therapy to work on his writing, but though the exercises helped a bit, no answer was found for the source of the problem. His joints throbbed and he took medications for pain but these only made him more comfortable, and did not cure him.

Pete was lucky because his pediatrician was a Lyme expert and this was only because she had Lyme once herself. She asked him if he had ever had a tick bite. Claudia, his mom remembered a day at the pool when she saw a tiny black dot on the back of his neck. Though she had removed the tick, three days later, a small red ring formed where the bite had been that was in the shape of a bull's eye. His tick bite formed a lump in the spring and fall. These are symptoms of Early Onset Lyme disease.

The perplexing situation for diagnosing Pete correctly was that though he had all the symptoms of Lyme, his test showed he was negative. His mother thought his bite at the time was strange and did not look right, so she took a picture. Because of this evidence, Dr. Smith tested several times in several different ways, finally insisting that Pete had Lyme.

Pete took several antibiotics to treat his Lyme disease. Dr. Smith gave him Doxycycline but when Pete tried this, he threw up almost instantly. Dr. Smith had to use a different antibiotic. Over time, she had to use several antibiotics like Minocycline, Bicillin an antibiotic injection, and Zithromax. Further tests showed he also had Rocky Mountain Spotted Fever and Babesia.

Pete already had constipation and diarrhea occasionally without a known cause but with all the antibiotics, he would throw up violently after breakfast sometimes and had a difficult time eating because the food made him feel sick. Dr. Smith had to give him many supplements to help repair his gut, and prevent further damage.

She gave him preventive antifungals like Diflucan and Nystatin because all those antibiotics made his gut worse and Candida in the gut. Further, he took extra vitamins that were not absorbed from his food correctly. He took a multivitamin, extra vitamin C and D, E, and cod liver oil and Cysteplus for his liver.

Pete had a medical, behavioral and school team to help him get through his ordeal. As the pain subsided he could write longer and get more down before he was in pain and his physical therapist gave him a pencil grip to tighten his grip on the pencil which reduced the pain in his hand. His Individual Education Plan (IEP) specified that he could type on the computer instead of write by hand when this was easier for him.

His anger and depression resolved unevenly at best, depending on his pain level and coping skills. He had a therapist to teach him what to do when he felt overwhelmed and frustrated. He had counselors at school to talk with when he could not cope and his teachers made contracts and plans with him to earn rewards when he finished his work on time.

After he was treated for Lyme for about a year or so, Pete began IVIG an IV treatment that would boost his immunity, with treatments two days in a row, once a month. The treatment itself was not particularly pleasant for him, but after five treatments, Pete went through a remarkable change in his behavior. He did not need the counselor to calm him down and instead he could calm himself. Small things did not bother him as much or as often. He even made friends.

His autism symptoms were mostly expressed in behavior issues, but the difference now was that he knew when he would feel anxious and could calm himself. He knew who he could talk with to regain composure when he needed help. He could explain how he felt and what bothered him.

His pain was less and his memory was better. He could thrive in the right environment.

Tools for Pete's Family
Although the treatment for Lyme is thirty days of antibiotics, some people need a more thorough examination and treatment to make sure the Lyme is truly gone.
If one family member has Lyme, test everyone. The mother can give it to her unborn child.[37]
It was clear that Pete's pain began soon after a tick bite. Some don't remember getting a tick bite, but if there are sudden changes in behavior after the tick bite along with flu like symptoms especially with the bull's-eye rash, this is Lyme.
As explained in Part 1 of this book (regarding the gut and immunity), when taking antibiotics, one must take care of the damage that can have on the gut. He had Bicillin an antibiotic that was injected to bypass this problem. Bicillin is a shot, however, and difficult if kids don't like shots. (Who does?)

Why Is Lyme Important?

Lyme presents with mental, physical and medical symptoms that can vary for everyone. If one member of your family has Lyme, there's a good chance others will have it as well, including your pets. Dogs and cats can bring an infected tick into the house.[38] The tests for Lyme are not as accurate as they once were and some people do not respond to treatment very well. Doctors do not test or diagnose for other diseases that ticks also carry unless they are what we call Lyme Literate, understanding the complexities of Lyme disease. Lyme is important to kids with autism because infectious diseases such as Lyme create a vulnerable immune system leading to an increased tendency for Autism Spectrum disorders in infancy and during fetal development.[39] The CDC estimates approximately 300,000 new cases of Lyme are diagnosed each year.[40] Additionally, new cases of Lyme are listed as an underlying cause of death in 114 cases from 1999 to 2003.[41]

What is Lyme?

Lyme borreliosis is an inflammatory blood borne disease transmitted by a black legged tick first discovered in Lyme, Connecticut, where children contracted rheumatoid arthritis in the 1970s.[42] Later in 1982, Willy Burgdorfer discovered the spirochetes reacting to the immunity of the patients who have Lyme. [43] Some studies indicate that it is also transmitted via mosquitoes. [44] Controversy exists on whether Lyme is sexually transmitted. Some studies say yes[45], while the CDC says no[46]. A controversial claim persists that Lyme began accidently at <u>USDA Research at Plum Island Animal Disease Center</u>. <u>The book *Lab257* by Michael Carroll</u> examines this theory. Other scientists suggest Lyme has been around for ages.

Symptoms

Approximately twenty to thirty percent of those with autism have Lyme disease.[47] In some cases, Lyme treatment improves the health and behavior outcomes of the child. Our family doctor, Warren Levin, MD (since retired) found twelve cases in a row of children with Lyme and autism. When he treated the Lyme disease, the autism symptoms decreased as well. He has always insisted that every child with autism get a definitive test for Lyme.

Lyme "The Great Imitator"

Lyme Disease will desecrate the immune system. It can sit in wait until another infection will manifest. Appendix F lists diseases such as MS, Fibromyalgia, and Chronic Fatigue Syndrome and compares their symptoms to Lyme. Sometimes, people with Lyme disease get misdiagnosed as having something else.

Physical Symptoms

The basic symptoms are joint pain, headache fatigue, fever and muscle pain similar to the flu. The CDC lists these as the most common symptoms.[48]

Mental Symptoms

Behavioral and emotional symptoms include depression, psychiatric, manic, and panic disorders, including Chronic Fatigue, Brain Fog, Cognition, Depression, and Dementia.[49]

Tests and Diagnosis

Sometimes, the tick bites in the hair, and therefore the bull's eye rash is not easy to spot. Many times people do not remember getting a tick bite, nor remember the rash. Also, the doctor must take every aspect of Lyme into account and make his own determination as to whether someone has Lyme disease.

Parents testing for Lyme need to be proactive with doctors, since diagnosis has been made more difficult by standardizing tests. Doctors attempted to standardize Lyme disease diagnosis and changed the way it was diagnosed in 1995 to rectify this confusion. This standardized test simply stated yes or no with no grey area and so it could miss people who had Lyme. Prior to 1994, the diagnosis of Lyme was done clinically combining with laboratory findings. After 1995, the new way was to attempt to standardize and to only look for specific markers, even if other markers were also indicators that one had Lyme disease. The testing should have been up to the doctor's discretion but instead the doctor could only report a positive or a negative finding and sometimes the results were not so crystal clear.[50]

After 1995, the Western Blot looked for specific bands and if any other bacteria besides the ones noted were found, they were generally ignored even if significant to the Lyme diagnosis. In 1995 under the new criteria 22 out of 66 patients were considered positive for Lyme at a Rheumatology Symposium. In the old criteria, all 66 would be positive.[51] When the diagnosis changed for Lyme that changes the criteria of how effective treatments work or if they work at all.[52]

Therefore, patients need to be certain they document tick bites and symptoms, and ask for wider interpretation of results, or work with a Lyme Literate doctor.

Vaccines

The new Lyme definition only defines it correctly in 15% of cases, which means that 85% get a negative test result even though they do have Lyme. This makes the Lymerix vaccine appear to be 85% more effective. However, the vaccine caused "Lyme-like symptoms" in those that had it when they were once healthy individuals.[53]

There was a class action lawsuit for this vaccine, by Sheller, Ludwig & Bailey filed against the Smith Kline Beecham, who represented 121 individuals who claimed they experienced significant adverse reactions including arthritis and "Lyme-like" symptoms.[54] Lymerix was taken off the market because of a lack of adequate sales.[55]

Ticks Carry More Than Lyme

Ticks carry other diseases besides Lyme, such as Babesia, Bartonella, Toxoplasmosis and Mycoplasma. Mycoplasma may be a contributor in 58% of those on the spectrum. Mycoplasma, Bartonella and Lyme are opportunistic infections, meaning they destroy the immune system, allowing the body to be vulnerable for an otherwise dormant symptomatic infection to become deadly.[56]

Babesia, a parasite that infects red blood cells and causes malaria, can be transmitted by a tick, from the mother to the unborn child and through blood transfusions. Symptoms are generally mild and start with a fever, muscle aches, chest and hip pain, shortness of breath, fatigue and headache. They are more severe for those with a weak immune system or no spleen. Babesia can be treated with anti-malaria drugs and antibiotics.[57]

Bartonella or cat scratch fever is a parasite that hides in red blood cells and causes fever, fatigue, headache, low appetite, swollen glands, and neurologic symptoms. Some symptoms also include marks that look like a scratch.[58]

Toxoplasmosis, a Lyme co-infection that comes from a parasite, can alter brain chemistry because it lowers dopamine levels. It also additionally creates a higher testosterone level. [59, 60] Dopamine is responsible for regulating reward behaviors including social interactions, appetite and addiction. [61] Doctors often correct lowered dopamine levels in those with Lyme without considering testing for Toxoplasmosis.

Mycoplasma Fermentans is a very tiny type of Mycoplasma that has no cell wall and depends upon the host to survive. Antibiotics don't eradicate this infection. The

CDC explains that Mycoplasma Pneumoniae is a bacteria lung infection, often called walking pneumonia. It is generally a mild illness like a chest cold with symptoms like a sore throat.[62]

According to the CDC, ticks also carry diseases such as Anaplasmosis, Babesiosis, Borrelia Miyamotoi, Colorado Tick Fever, Ehrlichiosis, Heartland Virus, Powassan Disease, Rickettsia Parkeri Rickettsiosis, Rocky Mountain Spotted Fever, Southern Tick Associated Rash Illness, Tick-borne Relapsing Fever and Tularaemia.[63]

Standard Lyme Treatment

What we consider standard treatment for Lyme may not be adequate. The CDC even says that after treatment, people may have Post Treatment Lyme Disease Syndrome, with ongoing symptoms. The CDC protocol is antibiotics such as doxycycline for 2 to 4 weeks.[64]

How to Avoid Tick Bites

Wear boots or long pants with socks if you decide to go hiking. Stay on the trails where there is less brush and plants where a tick might lurk. If you are in a place where you think ticks would be, do a tick check when you get home. If you find one try to preserve the whole tick because it's easier for the doctor to test the tick than to test you. If you remove the tick and it was broken into smaller pieces the tick cannot be tested. If you have the bull's eye rash, take a picture to bring with you to the doctor as a classic sign of Lyme disease.

Lyme Literate Doctors

If you suspect your child's autism is made worse by Lyme, you need a Lyme Literate doctor. This means a doctor that understands that ticks carry diseases other than Lyme, that these co-infections and sometimes mental symptoms can be included in the Lyme diagnosis. This doctor would know how to interpret the test results to diagnose Lyme accurately and even in some cases, testing more than once. The best type of Lyme literate doctor is one who has experienced Lyme himself. Here is a list of <u>Lyme Literate Doctors.</u>[65]

Tools for Dealing with Lyme Disease

Lyme is very common and can be a missing piece as to why your child's behaviors don't improve or why he doesn't feel better. Don't be afraid to ask your doctor repeatedly for Lyme testing especially if the child has a lot of fatigue, pain, and or is depressed.

Doctors will sometimes give psychiatric medications for behaviors. Because chronic Lyme can take years to correct, the treatments for Lyme may not show any direct effect on behaviors. These meds fix the chemical imbalance but the Lyme or its co-infections are the root. If this happens, find a Lyme literate psychiatrist. This doctor will understand the connections with Lyme and help you wean your child off the drugs. I would never recommend these types of medications but I know how the system works. Sometimes asking friends for referrals can help.

Refer to *Navigating the IEP* in Part 5, about services the school may offer if you ask.

You can ask for an aide, a behavior intervention plan, ABA therapy, or a psychologist or social worker to help your child out of a jam. Add these things to his IEP and make sure whatever he needs is written down.

When your child begins school, wait a few weeks and call the school to ask how he's doing and see if adjustments are needed.

These are tips to "get by" until you can treat the Lyme properly, which could take time.

Part 3: Toxicity: How does Environment Affect Behavior?

Nathan: The Personality Changer

When Nathan was a year old, he said his first words. "Turn the light on, please." He spoke a full sentence clear as day. When he was two, he was pointing at things, asking "What is this? What is that?" From the time, he could speak he named things and could ask for what he wanted.

He was a curious child. When he was three he began to build things, like intricate roadways for his Hot Wheels cars. He loved Legos and his mother, Beth, kept buying him kits. He had some cardboard bricks that he would build big towers just so he could knock them over. He had a play tent that had a post office slot on one side and on the other side it had a grocery store, where he "sold" things he'd take from the kitchen. He would draw pictures and tell his mom it was a letter she had to mail and she would put it in the pretend mail slot. When his brother was the postal carrier, he would stay inside the tent waiting for his letter to arrive. They would keep putting things in the mail slot saying they were mailing them but sometimes to see if they would fit.

Nathan's regression was slow and not so noticeable at first. He began to get blotchy rashes on his face, like eczema. Soon, Nathan was constantly sick with ear infections and fevers, and he always had a rash. His mother was told to give him Tylenol to break the fever. A few years later he had bronchitis and even scarlet fever. He had been to the doctor to rent a nebulizer to clear his lungs so many times that his parents ended up buying one, which cost several hundred dollars.

His words were garbled like he was drunk, for no apparent reason. He became difficult to understand and often screamed and became impatient when people didn't give him what he wanted because they could not understand him. He steadily lost consonants and began to give up. He was no longer interested in building things or playing post office.

Nathan began to exhibit some strange new behavior that was new to him. He liked to lie down with his stomach over the swing and spin around and around, until he couldn't spin anymore and then he would let go with his feet and literally unwind. He would do this repeatedly. When it was time to come inside, he would walk to the arm of the couch and lean onto the armrest. If he had to move away from the swing or the chair, he poked himself in the stomach.

He became obsessed with electronics and pressing buttons. He loved escalators, elevators and cash registers. When it was time to pay, he would walk over to the cash register and press every button changing the credit card machine to read in Spanish. He loved escalators and would want to go to the store and ride them up and down all day if he could. When he rode the elevator, he pressed every button, stopping at every floor annoying anyone who rode with him.

Nathan refused to eat anything other than seafood and cheese. Nathan loved fish, crab and oysters. He could drink a whole gallon of milk by himself. His doctor said that whole milk was good for his bones because it had calcium. He was very skinny and short for his age with a big round belly. When he ate, he was insatiable like he was always starving and had not eaten even when he had eaten ten minutes ago, "He must be made of cheese," Beth thought, watching him eat so much of it.

He walked around on his tip toes holding the wall sometimes for balance moving to the left and right, swaying a little bit as if the he was walking on a boat out at sea. He was always running to the bathroom because when he had to poop it poured out of him, like a faucet. His mother was always ready with a change of clothes, and knew where every bathroom was when they went out. Nathan wore pull-ups.

Nathan hated baths. He would scream so loudly his neighbor called the police several times. Nathan was very sensitive to the bath temperature and this was his only way to let his mother know. When the policemen came to the door, he heard Nathan say. "Hot! Hot! Hot!" Luckily, the policeman who came to the door had a child with autism and knew what Nathan had been experiencing, and left.

Nathan started preschool in a class full of other students with learning disorders including autism. Nathan had a difficult time asking for what he needed which led to frustration, tears and screaming. Sounds bothered him. Fire drills, balloons popping, fireworks, and music hurt his ears so he would hold his hands tight over them to shut out the noise. Sometimes he simply ran out of the room to escape.

He would become frustrated that his teachers at school did not understand him so he became louder and louder to make sure they heard him clearly. His energy and frustration built up throughout his day and he would have to release it by flapping his hands like a bird and running around and around in a circle repeating over and over hoping that someone would finally understand him, knocking over anything in his way.

Beth ultimately discovered that she had suffered from her own toxicity from mercury in her teeth and her yearly flu shot. She had Temporomandibular Joint Dysfunction (TMJ) that caused her jaw to crack and click. She always woke up with a headache that never really went away. She could not open her mouth all the way and sometimes chewing foods was difficult. She had been this way for decades before Nathan was born. Her jaw had a hole inside it called a cavitation, which is like a cavity in the teeth but in the jawbone. When she was in high school she had her wisdom teeth out and the hole remained. The mercury from her teeth stayed in this location causing a huge amount of pain for so long she felt like it was normal.

Nathan's mother studied the side effects of mercury and lead toxicity. Fatigue, headaches, joint pain which were her symptoms but also constipation, sound sensitivity and a loss of language which were Nathan's symptoms. She realized that she was also exposed because they both had symptoms even when they were both different. She not only had to detoxify Nathan but also for herself. She not only had to clear her house of mercury and lead, but also remove it from the body.

Nathan's family found out that their beautiful house was covered with toxins from the paint, to the old tub to the pipes. They lived within ten miles of a coal-fired power plant that leaked mercury into the air. The lead toxicity came from her water supply, and claw foot tub that contained lead as well as the old lead paint used throughout her house. She repainted and bought a water filter but still needed more money to redo her bathroom.

Nathan's doctor first tested Nathan's hair for metal toxicity and found nothing. Then he did a more thorough test called a porphyrin test. This test pulls the mercury out of his liver, kidney and brain to appear in a urine analysis. First, Beth collected Nathan's urine for six hours. Then she gave him EDTA a type of chelation that pulls out the mercury from the body, and then another six-hour urine collection. The test compares the before and after chelation which for Nathan showed a high quantity of mercury, aluminum and lead. His hair showed nothing because Nathan could not detoxify properly. If he could, the metals would show up in the hair. The post analysis of the chelation treatment showed huge amounts of metals in his urine showing that it was in his body, but not in his urine or his hair as it should have been if he was healthy.

When Beth started to research, she found that the mercury came from her teeth in her dental amalgams, which are black or silver fillings, the coal fired power plant that was within a few miles of her house, and from her flu shots. The lead came from the paint, and the pipes in her bathroom. The aluminum also came from other vaccines.

Beth's next step was to figure out where these metals came from and remove them as much as possible from their environment. She could not detoxify her own body without removing what was causing it. This means that she would have to remove the dental amalgams from her teeth, redo her bathroom to get rid of the lead pipes and get a water filter, and even move completely to avoid the coal fired power plants.

Nathan was born with his toxicity, because he was breathing in the mercury vapor from her teeth in utero, and exposed to mercury in the flu shot she had while pregnant. He had a Hepatitis B vaccine when he was first born, so he was also exposed to aluminum, and he took baths in water that contained lead.

Beth could not afford to move away from the coal fired power plants, but did eventually remove the dental amalgams from her teeth, repair the jaw cavitation and see a dentist for a mouth guard to correct her bite. She had also avoided the injected multi dose flu shots to prevent further mercury exposure.

Beth could not afford a water filter for her whole house, but did manage a water filter for cooking and drinking in the kitchen sink. She could not afford to redo her bathroom, but did some minimal repairs. She also bought Nathan a floating temperature gauge to test the water to get it the right temperature and that avoided some frustration.

Nathan went through many years of chelation therapy and a carbohydrate and sugar free diet. He wears noise-canceling headphones to drown out noise when things are too loud. He wears soft cotton clothes that are more comfortable. He does not speak in a traditional way but he still learned ways to get his point across.

His aide, Jane, was his translator, because although Nathan could not speak, he was communicating. When his shirt was too itchy, he took it off and brought a different shirt to his mom so she could help him get dressed. If he wanted cookies, he looked for them by opening the cabinets. Jane taught him some sign language, so that he could sign "cookie" instead of making a mess. Instead of screaming because the coffee maker was too loud, Nathan would put on headphones and turn off the coffee maker. His communication was clearer even with garbled words.

The headphones really helped him calm himself when noises were too loud. Beth and Nathan would watch videos together to learn how to sign. Once Nathan turned eight, he suddenly relearned that things had names and he could sign them. He picked up sign language quickly and learned new words faster than Beth could and sometimes he did not know the sign, but he made it up. Beth needed to learn to sign much faster to keep up with him.

Beth had to learn to sign as well if she wanted to talk to him. Eventually he learned to sign "loud", "hungry" and "thirsty." Beth learned the Standard American Sign Language and Nathan's made up sign language, but between the two, Nathan and Beth had learned how to communicate well without speaking.

For Nathan to cope with noises, bad tasting foods, or itchy clothes, he had to make these needs clear to those around him. He put his hands on his ears when things were loud, or took off his shirt when his clothes were itchy. He spat out the spicy foods. He needed to see pictures of different foods, so he could point to what he wanted.

Nathan's mother had to see detoxifying as a work in progress. With each coping skill, his behavior improved, and as Beth learned what to buy to ease the stress for Nathan he was less frustrated and more able to express his pain.

Sometimes autism is like a battlefield. Remove the war against uncomfortable clothes, spicy foods, and loud noises so that he can concentrate. Remove smelly items, and lower the volume, only then can Nathan begin to think clearly and feel peaceful and concentrate for better communication.

Tools for Nathan's Family

Identify any exposure to mercury before birth, using the porphyrin test.[66]. All the flu shots Beth had before and during pregnancy, eating fish, living near a coal fired power plant as well as the dental amalgams all contributed to his high mercury levels. She not only needed to detoxify from the metal exposure but not allow this to continue. This is an expensive ordeal and one that she had to figure out if it was financially feasible.

Here are some good tricks for picky eaters. Combining foods or mixing them in purees can help him expand his food choices, let him pick the menu, mix supplements in the smoothie, and add some real cheese with the cheese substitute and taper down slowly. If he must eat fish, be aware that the bigger the fish the more mercury it contains. Avoid farm raised and ask for wild caught fish if you must eat it at all.

Candida build-up: Candida or excess fungal infections in the gut can be increased by his food choices such as carbohydrates and sugar but also the antibiotics and metals. Often parents use an antifungal treatments and metals at the same time which is expensive and difficult on the body especially younger kids. Some parents have the money to do it all at once, but for the sake of a healthy child, it is necessary to slow it down and to do things at a pace his body can physically handle. Candida is a barrier to the metals, that's why there is excess when there is a lot of metals, but there may be behaviors as a result of either Candida or the metals or both.

Tylenol reaction: If Nathan cannot detoxify appropriately he should not take Tylenol, and never take Tylenol and a vaccine at the same time. If you cannot detoxify, the Tylenol only increases that effect, and the toxicity will only get worse.

Why Is Understanding Toxicity So Important?

We are born with an overwhelming toxic burden. "Of America's 73 million children, almost 21 million, nearly 1 out of 3 suffer from one chronic disease or another."[67] The toxic burden comes from generations of exposure, what you were exposed while pregnant and what your child's exposures are right now.

What your grandparents were exposed to can affect their genes and in turn affect your genes and your child's inheritance. Our children are one of the first generations to not live as their parents. Just because you have a gene does not mean that disease or disorder will manifest, because it all depends on whether that gene is expressed. Epigenetics is the external modification of DNA and whether gene expression is turned on or off.[68]

Researchers have been saying for the past decade that all autism was genetic primarily based on two factors. First, some children are born with autism. Second, they compared fraternal and identical twins for genetic versus environmental links.

There are problems with studying autism this way. Some kids have the genetics associated with autism which are either damaged because of toxicity or genes that create the inability to detoxify properly. Twins are not always the best way to study autism. There are environmental factors in common with twins because they tend to be preemies, it matters whether they are boys or girls or one of each, what the mother does while pregnant can affect both kids.

The inability to detoxify from our environment comes from mechanisms like methylation, and genes like APOE4 and MTHFR. The other genes that can become damaged from methylation include mitochondria dysfunction, SHANK3, and Tuberous Sclerosis.

Methylation has many functions. It affects whether you can detoxify appropriately, your energy level, your mood, and every cell in your body. Methylation is when a molecule passed a methyl group to make things like CoQ10 and melatonin and many others.[69] Methylation is responsible for epigenetics or the ability of whether of a gene is turned on or off.[70] There are also physical signs of unbalanced methylation issues, which are things like cancer, autism, chronic fatigue syndrome, dementia, diabetes, mood and psychiatric disorders.[71] You may have the genes for these issues but it still depends on how much you were exposed in the past, what your ancestors were exposed, and what you are exposed to right now.

There are lots of genes associated with autism. One key gene is Methyl Tetrahydrofolate Reductase (MTHFR), which is also an enzyme that has many functions and is associated with many diseases. MTHFR stabilizes DNA, regulates your hormones, mood, sleep, energy, detoxification, growth hormone, autonomic nervous system. MTHFR is responsible for making B12 and Folate. Without B12 you can't absorb the nutrients in your foods. 25% of kids on the spectrum have a mutation of MTHFR.[72]

Your energy and your sleep is also affected by methylation and MTHFR. Methylation regulates the production of ATP that gives your cells energy and it also affects mitochondria.[73] "In the autism community, 20% have an underlying mutation that puts them at risk for a mitochondrial dysfunction."[74]

Mitochondria are the battery of the cell, supplying vital energy. They can be damaged from metals, pharmaceutical medications, and chemical insults. Magnesium, Bicarbonate, Selenium, and Sulfur are important to the mitochondria to function optimally.[75] When pursuing the study of toxicology and chemical pollutants, there should be greater emphasis on the mitochondria.[76]

Some people may not know if they or their family members have mitochondrial disease or disorders but there are common symptoms. The United Mitochondria Disease Foundation lists: muscle control, gastrointestinal issues, seizures, cardio or liver disease, diabetes, respiratory distress, and vision or hearing issues. If these are in your family history, this potential is worth pursuing with your doctor. 50 million people have mitochondrial dysfunction, associated with other diseases such as Parkinson's, obesity, dementia, strokes and ALS.[77]

Methylation also affects your ability to generate glutathione, which helps the body detoxify appropriately. Glutathione is your body's shield to protect the liver, brain, heart and other organs from toxicity from many environmental sources including the mercury in multi-dose flu vaccines.[78]

Another gene that will prevent you or your child from removal of toxins is APOE. This is a housekeeping protein that can determine if an individual can excrete mercury. It moves from brain cells to the cerebral spinal fluid, to the blood and then the liver where it is excreted. There are three types, the APOE2, 3 and 4.

If you have the APOE2 gene, there are two binding sites where mercury can be excreted. The people with this type can have many exposures and many vaccines and are not as sick. They can smoke more with less chance for lung cancer or experience no side effects from dental amalgams in their teeth. Genes such as APOE2 are the reason why some can get vaccine or smoke a cigarette and not feel sick.

People with APOE3 can excrete some amount of metal so they may have some minor toxicity symptoms and may be able to handle some toxicity or perhaps are the ones who get some vaccines or delay them until later. They may handle some toxicity but not all. The problem for them is to not know how sick they would become from a vaccine or how many.

APOE4 gene-carriers are the people who should avoid toxicity as much as possible including vaccines. They cannot excrete at all.[79,80] Doctors do not normally check people for this gene before getting a vaccine or before we get a dental amalgam or buy a house with lead pipes. We do not know our toxicity level until we are exposed and become ill. **There are over 200 genes associated with autism that can create damage from toxicity.**[81]

Tuberous Sclerosis Complex is a genetic disorder where benign tumors to grow in the brain, or other organs such as the kidney or the heart. Symptoms result in behavior problems such as aggression, rage, ADHD, or obsessive compulsiveness. One third of those with TSC have symptoms of autism.[82] TSC will create seizures but the longer before the first seizure, the better. In one case in 1986, a DPT shot aggravated the seizure, reactivating the TSC. The child was compensated for the seizures but not for the autism.[83] Not all people with TSC will have overt symptoms.

You can also be born with toxicity. Researchers found an average of 200 industrial chemicals and pollutants in umbilical cord blood from 10 babies born in August and September of 2004 in U.S. hospitals. Tests revealed a total of 287 chemicals in the group including pesticides, consumer product ingredients, and wastes from burning coal, gasoline, and garbage. Those chemicals include 180 that are known to cause cancer.[84]

The gold standard for studying genetics is to study twins, but this method is not infallible because if twins are preemies, their sex, and the pregnant mother's medications and vaccines while pregnant will affect the health and well-being of her babies more.

Twins are more likely to be born premature than singletons, and whether they are male or female play a part in autism. Preemies or those babies born early are more susceptible to toxicity than a baby born on time. The CDC states that premature babies are a cause of neurological disabilities.[85] Whether twins are male or female is a predetermining factor for autism.[86] Twins could be one male, one female or one of each. Since autism is five times more common in boys, their sex is also an important criterion.[87]

We can be born with autism but that's because along with the genes already mentioned, and 200 more I haven't, sometimes the pregnant mother is already toxic or exposed to toxicity while pregnant. Dental amalgams, medications and lead are three ways pregnant women are exposed to toxicity before pregnancy or while she is already pregnant.

A video called *Toxic Teeth* from the International Academy of Oral Medicine and Toxicology explains that dental amalgams are the top source of human exposure to mercury and that any stimulation such as a dental cleaning, drinking coffee, chewing gum or grinding your teeth releases mercury vapor, which continues for an hour and half after the activity stops.[88]

Boyd Haley in a letter to Dan Burton explains the toxicity of dental amalgams. "Elemental mercury from dental amalgams could work synergistically with other ethyl mercury sources and have a cumulative toxic effect on the body. This could be the potential cause of autism and Alzheimer's disease."[89]

The American Dental Association considers dental amalgams to be "safe, durable and affordable,"[90] yet the Environmental Protection Agency states that dental clinics are the main source of mercury in Public Owned Treatment Works. 50% of mercury from POTW come from dental offices, and dental offices discharge 4.4 tons of mercury each year.[91] Both dental amalgams and multi-dose flu vaccines are considered hazardous waste[92] yet the CDC states that vaccines are safe and effective. For a complete understanding of the toxicity of Thimerosal in the multi-vial flu vaccines, please read Part 4: *Why Are Vaccines So Controversial?*

Lead exposure is found in paint, toys, your drinking water and painted furniture, Astroturf [93] and on the playground at school.[94] This is a good reason to monitor where and when your child has behavior problems. If there is toxicity where your child plays or where he learns, he may not reach his potential.

Mother's medications, such as Prozac and Zoloft (SSRIs), Terbutaline, and Tylenol, taken while pregnant can also make a child to be born with toxicity. These medications can make complications for both the mother as well as the baby and sets them up for toxic overloads.

Drugs to treat depression, if given to a pregnant mother, result in autism and birth defects in their children. Drugs such as Prozac, or Zoloft are SSRIs which stand for selective serotonin reuptake inhibitors causing autism in in the child in nearly twice as many cases as those who did not and nearly four times as likely if they took these medications in the first trimester.[95]

"Terbutaline was used off label for long-term management of preterm labor; such use is associated with increased risk of neurodevelopment disorders including autism spectrum disorders."[96] I mention this because I took it during my own pregnancy to prevent premature labor and consider this exposure as one of many associations of autism in my family.

The increased risk of autism, Asthma, and ADD also coincides with the replacement of aspirin with acetaminophen in genetically vulnerable children and in pregnant women. [97] Additionally, Acetaminophen or Tylenol increases the risk of autism as well if used with the measles mumps rubella vaccine in children five years old or less.[98]

Our toxicity is a cumulative build up. Our children are exposed to toxicity at home and at school. Often, when we test for toxicity, parents are not aware of where these might come from. Mercury, Lead and Pesticides will contribute to the toxic load as well. The method of exposure makes a difference on whether the body can remove it naturally.

The best strategy is to notice patterns of behavior among children if they happen in the same locations. You need to be a detective and use your common sense to figure out if toxicity is part of the problem, and if it's associated with a location.

How Does Toxicity Change Behavior? What does your child move towards or away from?

The child can sometimes be trying to communicate his toxic load if only we could see the cues. One child runs from a bad smell, holding his nose, or rips up a carpet sprayed with scotch guard, because he is trying to tell you that for him the carpet is toxic.

Some children are oblivious to the danger or even seem to gravitate towards it, as if they like the high they get from that smell or taste. Some have an IQ level that seems to drop quickly and just don't realize that danger is around them. Their parents have permanent two-year-old getting into everything, even when their adult child is 46. He smells his magic markers, runs into traffic, or eats the paste. We also know lead lowers the IQ levels in children.[99]

Here are some questions to ask when trying to resolve this in your child.

- Why does he do the same behaviors every time he's at the same location?
- What did he touch, taste or smell that could cause a reaction?

Physical symptoms give us clues to toxicity.

There are also physical symptoms that manifest with behavior that together give us clues. A child who has seizures at a funeral home, a construction site and his grandmother's house may be offering a clue to his medical problem. One mother found that formaldehyde was present in all three locations, even grandma's house because she used plug in air fresheners.

Children may know something is inherently wrong with the way their bodies function. They may not like the way it feels or know that there is something in their environment that is causing their pain so they will bite, scratch or simply run to get out of that environment. Appendix G includes physical and emotional signs of toxicity.

If your nonverbal child has these physical symptoms, here are some behaviors that might communicate his pain and offer you clues. If the child has red ear lobes and ear pain and is pulling on their ear lobes or holding their hands on their ears, that can be his way of telling you information about his ears but also telling you to do something about it.

A child who rubs his nose upwards, has nose wrinkles and runny nose and by constantly wiping, pinching or picking his nose, he may be telling you nonverbally there is something wrong with his nose.

A child who has wrinkles below the eyes, puffiness or under eye circles might be constantly rubbing his eyes, keeping his eyes closed or blinking often or running into things because he can't see or he may have an issue with his eyes like eye tearing or tracking.

A child with swollen puffy lips, puffy or red cheeks may be holding his hands over his mouth or moving his lips with hands to tell you that they hurt.

A child with constipation might run into the bathroom and sit on the toilet for hours even fully clothed. He may even squat in the corner. Sometimes if the child does not know where to go but has diarrhea might just be running to go to the bathroom, or not know where the bathroom is. He's basically constantly running. He may strip off his clothes because he has soiled himself and does not like the way it feels.

A child with a severe migraine may bang his head on the floor or the wall, or turn off the lights that are too bright, or put his hands on his ears when people are too loud.

Toxicity changes behavior in schools, prisons and for mental patients. A school in Wisconsin supported a complete change in student behavior just be switching their foods.[100] Tests on prisoners indicated excessive manganese, copper and mercury levels.

Additionally, toxicity including high lead, manganese, copper, or mercury is linked with ADHD, attention impulsivity, anger, aggression, inability to inhibit inappropriate responses, juvenile delinquency, and criminality. Mercury has been found to be a factor in anger, aggressive behavior, depression, obsessive-compulsive behavior (OCD), ADD, autism, schizophrenia, suicidal behaviors, learning disabilities, anxiety, mood disorders, and memory problems. Excess copper makes children behave violently.[101]

Places to Start

1. Parents' occupations

Do the parents have a job that has high toxicity exposures? I have listed in Appendix H some top occupations that have high toxicity exposures. Just because you work in one of these fields does not mean you will have a child on the spectrum. But if you do, the toxicity might be contributing as with vaccines and gut problems. I would point out that dentists are on that list. They are at risk for mercury vapor exposure leading to neurological insults.[102]

2. Schools and Homes

Both school and homes use the same unhealthy toxic products and one needs to be aware of where are when these occur to notice a pattern of physical, educational or behaviors that emerge when children or adults are in the same locations or perhaps during the same time of year when toxicity is likely to be present. This includes things like synthetic carpets, cleaning products, cigarette smoke, pesticides, or things containing lead like the water supply. Astroturf also contains lead that get stuck on the clothes or hair.[103]

Steps that can help

You can't clean up the whole world where your child lives. You cannot ask neighbors or relatives to stop smoking or avoid air fresheners, but parents do the best they can to keep their child's environment safe. Here are some practical tips about where to begin.

Medical tests can determine what toxicity is the most problematic. Start there.

I have given you a dramatic list of toxicity that feels as though it's everywhere all the time, but that doesn't mean that all these chemical contaminants are bothering your child. If your child's mercury level is off the charts, then mercury toxicity is where you begin, by avoiding all exposures. Whatever his biggest reaction is, that's your biggest obstacle. Your child may not react to all these toxic chemicals so as you organize your budget to clean up his environment, figure out his exposures and avoid them.

Kids who are chronically ill cannot learn.

Our kids are the canaries in the coalmine. They are too sick to learn at school, staying home with colds that may be allergies or toxic exposures at the school that are making them sick. Parents will pull the children out of school because the chemicals used within cause seizures, headaches or pain. Some children cannot learn in that environment at all or the damage is too great. Options include home schooling for even a year or two to give the kids time to heal, moving to a new school that has a better environment, or permanently staying home.

A friend of mine had a son who had up to 80 seizures a day. If your child is this challenged, you may be the parent who skips invitations, birthday parties or family reunions because leaving the house means your child could have yet another seizure. For these parents, you will always need an at home nurse, babysitter, or an aide to help you.

Social Media is your lifeline.

Parents are the experts because the doctors are lagging in research. Doctors risk their whole careers for simply questioning vaccines or searching for autism treatments. If you can't leave your house because your child's toxicity has reached such a tragic level, that does not mean you are shut out from the world. Instagram, Facebook, and Twitter are all your friends. Start a blog, a video channel, a website and share what you know. Whatever worked for your child to alleviate even just one symptom, or taught him a coping skill, or helped others to understand your child, sharing these things can save a life. Even just documenting your day in a diary can help someone go through the process of helping their children. Sometimes we just need moral support.

Skype or Facetime your friends

Friends that you can't travel to see are only a Facetime or a phone call away. Make that an option and reach out to each other. You don't have to be stuck in your house alone. You really do have friends and they care about your child. As soon as you share your story, people will share theirs too.

Impacts of Toxicity

Toxicity impacts education, absenteeism, standardized tests, poor children, obesity, learning, and budget cuts. We must remove toxicity not just from home but also from schools. All the toxicity is causing lower test scores, more drop outs, more absenteeism, autism, ADHD. We test and retest and fire teachers, cutting great programs like band or even recess because school administrators can't understand why the kids are not learning. The poor buy older houses that contain lead pipes, and get more vaccines than wealthier parents. We lose funding for art and music to make more room in the budget for therapists, disciplinarians, or for those with special needs. We make the exhausted child run laps when he needs to rest, and the obese kid starve, instead of teaching them how to eat better such as eating less MSG and GMOs. We tell kids who can't detox to play on Astroturf soccer fields that contain lead that can be in their shoes, clothing and hair, just so they can play in the rain. The true education that needs to be done is to teach our school administrators about toxins in the school. By removing them from the school environment, we get more education in less time and less effort. We can add more extracurricular things to the budget and more kids will be at school on time because they were not in pain.

Complications: An Autism Team that Doesn't Understand.

Finally, our autism teams are too specialized. The therapists only see things as behavioral. The doctors only see the symptoms. The psychologist or psychiatrist only sees a problem as a chemical imbalance or behavior that must be corrected, instead of asking how or why that behavior is happening medically and what the child is trying to tell us about his environment. His mood is better with less lead. The chemical imbalance is restored by not eating GMOs. He can focus on his studies without the distractions of overstimulation of noise. There are answers, if we only listen, and when we start to find the right solutions, we need the whole team to communicate and work together.

How Do We Make Our Children Healthy Again?

Toxicity must be removed physically from the child's environment while she heals. There are many things you can do to understand your child's toxicity. Study your family history before vaccinating and understand toxic loads. Keep a list of any medications given while pregnant including the number of vaccines as well as dental amalgams. Once you have tested for toxicity, find out if the child is currently exposed including school or home. Pay attention the physical symptoms, the behaviors, and the locations where the child was. Retrace his steps to find the toxicity. This can be difficult.

Toxicity Tests

Perhaps the most important test we need to do is for metals. The problem is that our kids are not detoxifying the way they are supposed to be. The metals are supposed to excrete through the hair, blood and sweat but instead the metals go to organs such as the kidney brain, and liver. The tests here are just a sample of tests your doctor may require. This is in no way a complete list of tests your doctor may ask of you or your child. I'm only listing a few to simplify because this can be overwhelming.

Porphyrin test. -This is a test that will show damage from toxic exposure, burden of toxicity and of drugs, and the before and after of chelation therapy.[104]

DMSA: This is a product to remove heavy metal toxicity. Often the doctor use the Porphyrin test, use the DMSA and then do the test again to pull the metals out of the body. There are many ways to do chelation, and this is by no means the only one.[105]

OAT stands for Organic Acid Test, used to evaluate intestinal yeast and bacteria.[106]

Ways to Help the Body Repair Itself

The body is supposed to heal itself when it is exposed to something that should not be there. Here are ways to encourage the body to Repair Itself:

- Clay bath
- HBOT
- Infrared sauna
- Ionic foot bath
- Epsom salts
- Product to remove glyphosate
- Essential oils
- Homeopathy
- Heal the damage
- Boost Glutathione
- Boost Immunity

Pay attention to physical and behavioral symptoms and where and when they occur.

Teach the teachers, the school board, and the board of supervisors how and why their policies are impacting education.

Part 4: Why are Vaccines So Controversial?

Jacob: The Threat

Thirteen-year old Jacob was a threat to himself and his own parents. He tried to strangle his baby brother, he accused his mom of poisoning him and if given the opportunity, his family feared he might go through on his plans to shoot himself in the head. His father had a gun, and although Jacob had no idea where his father kept the bullets, he had already threatened them with the unloaded pistol.

His parents were at a loss to explain his sudden violent tendencies and demands for everything. He thought his parents were drugging him and there were drugs in his water. He felt like he was floating above his body, as if he wasn't aware of his surroundings, and he was somewhere else.

After watching a movie about zombies, he had somehow dreamed that they were the cause of his misery. His father looked like the familiar forty-something bearded man that he knew to be his dad, but he sometimes also "knew" it wasn't "really" him. When Jacob imagined his father to be a zombie who was going to eat him. Jacob sometimes rubbed his eyes as his fantasy life and real life blurred together. He knew all those things weren't real. He just couldn't think clearly.

Jacob had all his vaccines on schedule but the DTAP always gave him issues. After the first DTAP, he had a seizure almost as soon as he got home. His doctor said he had epilepsy, but he had never had a seizure before that shot. Even though she knew better, his mother gave him his second DTAP because she thought he could not go to school without it. She was scared, though, because she also knew if he had another seizure it might kill him.

Jacob sometimes had blackouts where he would wake up dizzy and disoriented with drool on his chin. His parents said he had a seizure but he had no recollection of that, just a massive headache and a sore body, like he had the hardest workout of his life. He would wake up in a Hospital and had no idea how he got there. "Must be the zombies," he thought.

His doctor said there must be epilepsy in the family even though there clearly was not. Jacob had no history of seizures until the DTAP vaccine. His head hurt so bad that he wanted to die and he wanted so badly to understand how he got this way. He felt out of touch with the ground and was unaware of what was happening around him. He also knew that he was different after that shot.

His moments of clarity were about his new career goal to be a movie director. The movie he wanted to direct, of course was about zombies because they had become his obsession. He said, "My head feels like zombies are eating my brain." His head felt like parts of his brain were missing.

His head hurt too much to take a shower or bother getting dressed. His therapists told him not to push on the side of his head and they used ABA to stop him from doing it, but this pressure was a small relief to the pain he felt. His therapists made him learn to dress himself anyway and still go to school and learn things even when his head felt like half his brain had been devoured already.

Jacob went to an autism school especially designed for tough cases like him because they had physically powerful aides who could subdue him if needed. They were protecting him from himself. Jacob could communicate when he was calm and sometimes he did have a good day, but others he was tough and mean and angry. One thing that calmed him was the pacing that he did. It was a stimming behavior that soothed him when things got to rough, so his "bodyguards" had to give him a little walk to cool off, a release Jacob, even in his angriest state, enjoyed.

Walking was the only way he could think clearly, but in school you are supposed to sit down and be quiet. His teachers couldn't handle him and would put him a Seclusion Room used to calm people down. It was a small room with no windows, where he was supposed to "think about his actions." He would constantly get in trouble for getting out of his chair and walking around in circles because the room was the size of a small closet and not a good place to walk the way he wanted. He needed to vent, to breathe, to talk to someone and not be isolated.

When he did go on a walk, math problems became clearer, and he had great ideas about how to write his essays. He still had a hard time getting them on paper because of his gigantic headache. His teachers yelled to listen and pay attention but they just sounded like Charlie Brown's teachers with the volume turned up, a lot of noise and nothing to say. School was oddly boring; Jacob was smart and could read interesting things at home for fun but saw no real-life use for anything he was learning at school. They were telling the kids the right way to fill in the little circles for the Standards of Learning Test he would soon have to take. "Duh, anyone knows how to fill in a stupid circle. Can't we learn anything remotely interesting?"

When he was six, Jacob was diagnosed with Autism and only now in his teens they found that he had acute dissimilated encephalitis, which means inflammation of the brain. He had nerve damage in his feet and legs and sometimes the pain felt like someone stabbing him with a hundred steak knives. His brain was developing antibodies against itself, as if it was like a little zombie. He didn't know how to tell anyone that his head felt like a bomb had gone off in his skull so instead he would break things and destroy tables or chairs or anything that was big enough that he could throw.

Tools for Jacob and his Family

Until Jacob could learn the proper communication to explain to his parents, his obsession with zombies was really about his headache. He couldn't explain it logically, so he just seemed odd to the people around him. As in the definition of autism, our kids have trouble with communication and trying to understand what's wrong. His zombie obsession was his creative way of explaining it even if no one understood.

Jacob and his family had to go through numerous specialists and tests to find out he had encephalitis. He went to neurologists, developmental pediatricians, psychologists, and therapists for physical, occupational, and speech problems. He even went to an infectious disease specialist before he found the right treatment. When doctors could not find the proper diagnosis, they thought he was making it up, since the things he said sounded crazy. His parents thought the anger was part of his personality until they identified his high white blood cell count and decided to look deeper. The source of a behavior is not always part of their personality, but it takes effort and sometimes a lot of money to figure out if there is a medical condition causing the behaviors.

Encephalitis is autoimmunity, meaning his brain was attacking itself as if it was a foreign object. The part that it was attacking was related to emotions and executive functioning so therefore he had a hard time making rational decisions and why he was so angry.

Jacob had already had a seizure with his first DTAP vaccine. Someone who has already been injured by a vaccine does not need to be injured again. Encephalitis is a side effect of the vaccine he had, and a very serious one. Jacob did not need that vaccine if it was going to create such severe damage. In this case, the risks clearly outweigh the benefits and Jacob medically was not able to handle anymore. His mother didn't understand that each state has exemption policies and his parents had to follow the correct ones for his state.

In Jacob's case the damage to his brain was severe and not fixable. For the rest of his life, Jacob would always have seizures. His doctors could still treat the pain, though, which would reduce the anger.

Jacob's anger was a frustration that he was in pain and didn't know how to tell anyone or what to do about it. Improvement of communication to express his emotions can help and someone to carefully watch him for seizures. Some kids get IVIG who are like Jacob. Jacob is a difficult case not just for the anger but also for the seizures. His school environment needs the medical and physical support to handle both. Kids like Jacob may end up home schooled with an aide or an alternative program that offers both.

Jacob could now write down all the stories in his head because he no longer suffered from the headaches. You can guess what he wrote about: Zombies. This was his way of coping with what had happened to him and now he could express it creatively. Jacob had found a way to communicate with the written word and even though he needed his iPad to explain himself, he could now tell people what he needed which was a huge step. Jacob's grades improved when he was not in pain.

Jacob was not at all cured. He was managed or handled because he learned to cope with his toxic environment. Jacob was sensitive to smells and touch and those things were painful. Someone with a strong perfume or air freshener could give him a headache and even another seizure. His aides also helped him speak out and tell others what happens when these chemicals were around him. He was always going to be sensitive to chemicals which seemed to be everywhere, but he was also the strongest advocate to teach others what they were doing to themselves by using them. Jacob wasn't going to change everyone's mind but he had friends now and they complied with his requests, so he was able to build stronger relationships.

Frequently Asked Questions About Vaccines

Parents frequently hear the same statements about vaccine safety and effectiveness from schools, in the media and from their doctors. This part addresses all the common questions and answers your doctors or your friends might ask or report about vaccines. I have changed the format to address these common statements so that it helps you know what to say to defend your decisions when these come up in every day conversations. Your doctor may have been taught in medical school that vaccines are safe, when to give them out, and how, but he's not taught what's in the vaccine or to read the insert. Parents with vaccine injured kids, have done their homework.

This and the next part show the malfeasance of the CDC, demonstrating that they have not presented to the public, or to physicians, all the information you need to make the right decisions for your family. Vaccines are all about informed consent. The doctor by law must give you all the information to make the proper decisions about your health. Without this information, he has not done this.

Here are the most common statements:

- Vaccines are safe and effective.
- Immunized and vaccinated mean the same thing.
- Outbreaks are always because of people who skip or delay vaccines.
- Vaccines protect you from disease forever, thus creating the term "vaccine preventable."
- They tell parents that we must achieve herd immunity for vaccines to be effective.
- They dismiss your injuries as a coincidence.
- Every disease that has a vaccine is deadly and highly contagious.
- The vaccine must have "worn off" if you get the disease right after the vaccine.
- Tylenol is good to prevent a fever after a vaccine.

What is the Foundation for Vaccine Decisions?

As with all Medications, vaccines should be studied independently by a third party who does not benefit or profit from their use. Coleen Boyle, a doctor under oath representing the CDC states that there has never been an unbiased vaccinated vs. unvaccinated study.[107, 108] Vaccines are not studied against saline a true placebo, but against another vaccine with similar ingredients.[109] Those methods are questionable. Are the vaccines safe and effective? What do the experts say? That depends who you ask.

Parents should have the rights and responsibility to decide for themselves whether they or their children need a vaccine and when they want to get one. Patients should be responsible for their own healthcare and the people who give out the vaccines along with the manufacturers who make them should take responsibility if something should go wrong. No medication or surgery is infallible. [110] Surgeons make mistakes. Doctors do as well. No one should be forced against their will to comply with vaccines, especially if they might harm that individual.

There are some simple things parents can do to become informed so they can be comfortable with their decisions and take control of their child's vaccine protocol. Explore your vaccine facts not just one vaccine at a time but one manufacturer at a time. The flu mist has different side effects, different ingredients and for a different population than the other injected flu shots therefore you cannot just simply compare any specific vaccine for any one disease without naming which one you mean.[111,112] Doctors will tell you that these side effects are rare if they tell about them at all. The CDC says that the adverse events are only minor such as a sore arm or low-grade fever.[113]

It is important to take control of your medical needs because, as I will demonstrate, vaccines can be associated with "autism-like features," allergies, asthma, and sometimes other chronic disabilities. The stories included in this book are about medically treatable issues that happen right after a vaccine, but your doctor might see them as a coincidence. They also may be overlooked because if your child is nonverbal he can't you tell what's wrong.

What is the Difference between "Immunized" and "Vaccinated"?

These two words are often used interchangeably but if you can still get the disease they are two different things. The Webster Dictionary says immune means "not capable of being affected by a disease."[114] The CDC uses the words immunized and vaccinated to mean the same thing but they are not.

There are many boosters in the CDC's vaccine schedule, which means the CDC knows that the vaccine does not protect everyone all the time. There are outbreaks in the vaccinated populations, and that is proof that some vaccines do not always work as they were intended. When an outbreak of any disease occurs, one must investigate whether those with a vaccine preventable disease include a vaccinated population. If the vaccinated are sick, the vaccine did not prevent it.

Those who skip or delay vaccines often do so because they cannot be vaccinated or they have a sibling or family member with vaccine injuries. Most believed in vaccines and trusted them until something went wrong and began to search for answers. Vaccine injuries and immune deficiencies are common in the same family, so that when one child in a family dies from a vaccine-related injury, his younger sister has the right to refuse vaccines for herself. When states force vaccines, that little sister must choose between possible injury like her brother or attending school. That is no choice at all.

Ohio State University had an outbreak of 116 cases of mumps in which 113 were vaccinated, and had the mumps anyway. The spokesperson from the Columbia Health Department, Mr. Jose Rodriguez even emphasizes that the vaccinated are still at risk for catching mumps. "At least three of the infected people are confirmed as not having received vaccinations for the mumps. If even one person is unvaccinated we are all at risk,"[115]

The media emphasizes the three people who were not vaccinated without considering that most the people in the story were vaccinated and still contracted the mumps. That means the vaccination failed because they should have been protected but were not. It is your right as a consumer of vaccines to always ask how many people were vaccinated and still got sick during an outbreak. Why do I say this?

The Ohio story is about mumps spreading in a vaccinated community, yet the unvaccinated were to blame. The real reason the vaccinated still had the mumps was because there was a lawsuit alleging that the mumps portion of the MMR was ineffective. Two scientists are suing Merck, the manufacturer of the MMR, for fraud because the mumps vaccine had a poor efficacy.

The suit alleges. "As the single largest purchaser of childhood vaccines (accounting for more than 50 percent of all vaccine purchasers), the United States is by far the largest financial victim of Merck's fraud. But the ultimate victims here are the millions of children who every year are being injected with a mumps vaccine that is not providing them with an adequate level of protection against mumps.[116]

This is a pro-vaccine article that still shows the Mumps portion of the MMR is ineffective and yet every time there is an outbreak of Mumps doctors fail to mention it. The Mumps vaccine is still being used and parents are still blamed ridiculed and humiliated for refusing to be vaccinated with a vaccine that does not work as advertised.

Another vaccine that is not as effective as claimed is the flu vaccine. The Lancet published an analysis to state that Influenza vaccines only protect 1.5 out of 100 people in a metadata analysis of over 5,707 articles and 31 studies.[117]

Doctors will always claim that one shot is better than no shots at all but from this data, this is just barely so.

If you read the vaccine inserts, some vaccines use another vaccine as a placebo in experiments. That's like checking your alcohol level with a beer by measuring against a glass of wine. It's not a true placebo. Flulaval research used another flu vaccine, Fluzone, as a placebo.[118]

A placebo should be an inert substance like water or saline that measures what the patient perceives as a cure, to the actual medication that is being tested. You can't use a control too like a placebo and get an accurate result. This is elementary science. I don't need a Ph.D. in immunology to understand that this does not prove whether this vaccine works.

These examples illustrate that you can no longer just blame the unvaccinated for spreading disease. They are examples that call into question whether the vaccine works and the studies used to prove it. It also means that you can no longer interchange the words vaccinated and immunized because they mean two different things.

What is the Problem with "Herd Immunity"?

Herd immunity is the idea that if most people are vaccinated per the CDC schedule then the small amounts who are not vaccinated will also be protected from a disease.

There is a lot of hypocrisy when doctors, senators, school administrators, or other parents tell you that your child must have their vaccines to achieve herd immunity, yet these very same people don't get the same vaccines for themselves or their children. This is the case of saying one thing and doing another.

Children go to the mall, or the grocery store around people who are supposed to be deathly ill. Their teachers, even their doctors may be vaccinated per their age, but have only had a handful of vaccines as compared to kids. These people may be up to date, but that depends how old you are, and which date you mean.

When we say, we are "up to date" on our vaccines; we never are because there are always more to add to the schedule. There are more boosters added no matter how many the children have had that did not prevent disease the first time, even mandating that we take them. Wouldn't it be more responsible for the health and well-being of humanity to evaluate the effectiveness of vaccines and to access how many in the vaccinated population were sick? The adult population is next in line to get more vaccines added to the schedule. However, the vaccines that are not protecting the children will not protect the adults either. We need to change the paradigm of what we use to protect ourselves from disease because in some cases we are vaccinating ourselves to death.

The quantity of vaccines given out has become out of control because the CDC vaccine schedule is a living document that is constantly changing. More vaccines are added every day. We get the same vaccines repeatedly and yet there are still outbreaks. The CDC schedule says that children get 46 doses before the age of six.[119] In *The Greater Good* movie, they specify 70 doses of 16 vaccines by age 18. In 1983 there were 23 doses of 8 vaccines by age 18.[120]

We will keep giving vaccines, knowing they do not protect, because we are still afraid of catching a disease. The definition of insanity is doing the same thing repeatedly and expecting a different result. The example I will use is DTAP.

For just one vaccine, the DTAP we are given six vaccines before age twelve and one every ten years after that.[121] If you live to be 72 years old, that's twelve vaccines for the same diseases in your lifetime. The Cleveland Clinic admits that in two to three years, the efficacy for DTAP is 34% and this waning protection is the reason more adolescents get pertussis.[122] Even vaccinating every two years in your lifetime will still not achieve herd immunity or even offer you 50% protection.

Not all professionals believe in Herd Immunity. Russell Blaylock, a neurosurgeon has this to say about herd immunity. That vaccine-induced herd immunity is mostly myth can be proven quite simply. When I was in medical school, we were taught that all the childhood vaccines lasted a lifetime. This thinking existed for over 70 years. It was not until relatively recently that it was discovered that most of these vaccines lost their effectiveness two to ten years after being given.[123]

The public are no longer buying this idea that vaccines last a lifetime because the CDC quietly keeps adding more and more boosters to the schedule and mandating that people get them. The public is no longer afraid when there are a few isolated cases of a disease because if they truly believed in the faith of vaccines they would know they don't need more shots because they are already protected. Instead, drug stores offer loads of incentives to give you your vaccine and spend more on advertising. They even give you a discount which you can spend on the medications that you are not supposed to need because you were vaccinated.

The CDC is at the beginning of mandating vaccines state by state and even nationally with California as first in line. California has a bill SB277[124] to forcibly vaccinate children to attend school. They are also mandating vaccines for adults with SB792.[125] Clearly the vaccines are not lasting a lifetime and people are not lining up to get them or these mandates would not be necessary. There is also a pending bill, nationally HR2232 which mandates all vaccines for children in all fifty states.[126]

I will give three examples where a doctor on television or a host of a television show has promoted vaccines but either did not get vaccines for themselves or had had dire consequences when he did. Why promote vaccines on television, but not get them yourself? This is quite hypocritical.

Paul Offit has only had 4 vaccines, yet he says babies can tolerate 10,000 vaccines at once.[127] Piers Morgan was deathly ill after he had the flu vaccine on television. Dr. Nancy Snyderman did not follow her own advice when she went to Liberia after being exposed to Ebola.

When Dr. Paul Offit, an infectious disease specialist at the Children's Hospital of Philadelphia, was asked about how many vaccines he has had compared to children on an episode of Frontline he said:

"I was born in 1951. I got the smallpox vaccine. I also got the diphtheria and pertussis and tetanus vaccine. And then in the mid-1950s, I got Jonas Salk's inactivated polio vaccine. And that was it."[128] That's a total of 5 vaccines. Children now usually get 70 before age 18. Everyone knows 5 does not equal 70, and yet both children and adults like Dr. Offit are considered up to date.

The Department of Health in Minnesota, states that 70-90% of adults who don't remember getting chicken pox are naturally immune.[129] That means even if he never had chicken pox, he was exposed as a child and now he could be fully protected without ever being sick. Adults are not vaccinated the way kids are. Dr. Offit, because of his age, can test his antibodies for disease by taking a titer test. That sounds great for him, but parents who do this are kicked out of doctor's offices because they refuse to vaccinate their kids when they might be naturally immune by taking the same test.

Dr. Mehmet Oz gave Piers Morgan a flu shot live on television. Dr. Oz says that you cannot get the flu from a flu shot because it is a dead flu virus.[130] He says that getting the flu after the flu shot is a myth. Yet three weeks later Piers had the flu two times. Morgan noted, "He never had the flu until he had the flu shot."[131]

Dr. Nancy Snyderman, when asked about Ebola said, "We have a sophisticated health care system to isolate the patient and prevent further spread."[132] Later, after traveling to Liberia to help with the Ebola epidemic, she was seen at a favorite restaurant near her home, violating her quarantine to stay home after possible exposure.[133] "As a health professional, I know we have no symptoms and pose no risk to the public," she said.[134] If you go on TV to promote vaccines, and ask others to be under quarantine, the very least you can do is stay home because it makes the media look like they do not follow their own advice. Ebola petered out before the vaccine in Sierra Leone,[135] so in this case we cannot give the vaccine the credit. This article still promotes the vaccine even after Ebola is already gone.

We will keep vaccinating even by force to achieve herd immunity that does not exist and never has from a vaccine. Instead let's use a real saline placebo, let's test the whole vaccine schedule together, and let's have true informed consent. These pundits promoting vaccines would be the first to stop them if they knew what they were promoting and were not paid for doing so.

Is the Vaccine Schedule Safe?

There is important information to understand if you want to measure vaccine safety. What is the timing of the disease, vs. the timing of the vaccine? We should study the entire vaccine schedule not one vaccine at a time or even one disease at a time.

Vaccines are now studied one at a time, not as an entire schedule. I have established that vaccines wear off over time, so we should be checking when the vaccine was given as compared to the likelihood to get the disease.

The timing of the vaccine compared to the timing of when you catch the disease is also important. Hepatitis B is contracted from IV drug use, sex, or mother to baby, through bodily fluids.[136] Unless your baby is a drug user or sexually active, it would make more sense and prevent Hepatitis B in the baby if we test the mother. If the mother does not have it, neither does the baby. These mothers are accused of neglect because they refuse a vaccine given within hours of birth that is unnecessary.

If we can conclude there is no relationship between vaccines and autism, how do we know that baby has no autism when he is merely hours old when he gets his first vaccine? In fact, A 2010 study showed that boys were given the three hepatitis B vaccines starting a birth were three times more likely to develop autism than those that were never vaccinated.[137]

If vaccines are safe and effective, why have we not done a study to compare the vaccinated vs. those who refuse vaccines? Dr. Paul Offit believes you cannot do a vaccinated vs. unvaccinated study because it is unethical. He believes in the power of vaccines so strongly that it is unethical and immoral to not vaccinate. When he was on Frontline he said." Well, there are certain things about vaccines that are absolute truths. One is that they work. And if you choose not to get a vaccine, you are at greater risk of developing a disease [that] can cause you to suffer or be hospitalized and die. And if you have a large enough cohort of children who are vaccinated or unvaccinated, you can bet that there will be children in the unvaccinated group who will suffer that consequence. And no Institutional Review Board, and frankly no ethical researcher, could ever do that study, because you know that you have frankly condemned those in the unvaccinated group -- some in the unvaccinated group -- to develop diseases which can permanently harm them and/or kill them. You can't do that study."[138]

Occam's Razor is a scientific principle that is often ignored by scientists who promote vaccines. This theory states that the simplest explanation is usually correct.[139] If a car hits you, your broken leg from the car accident is not a coincidence. Doctors do not apply this logic to vaccine injuries. Vaccine injuries listed in the insert are considered a coincidence.

Children's vaccine side effects are only monitored for a few days after a vaccine and anything after that is a separate event. Adverse events for adults include anaphylaxis, allergies, seizures, inflammation of the brain or encephalopathy and Guillain-Barre, where the immune system attacks your nervous system,[140,141] yet if these same symptoms are shown in children who get seventy doses as compared to less than ten for adults, it's a coincidence. Dr.

Boyd Haley says, "A single vaccine given to a six-pound newborn is like giving a 180-lb. adult 30 vaccines on the same day."[142]

We can apply the same idea of correlation does not equal causation to the aspect of when and where you catch the diseases. Appendix I is a graph that shows three main components. There was no vaccine for typhoid, yet that disease incidence decreased at the same as the others because of good sanitation and better hygiene. Also, the point at which Polio, Small Pox, and Diptheria vaccine were introduced, these diseases all went down at the same rates. They all dropped before the vaccine began but we give the vaccine the credit.

Compulsory Vaccination, Vaccination A Curse and a Menace to Personal Liberty (1900), by JM Peebles, explained what it was like when there were diseases like The Plague or Smallpox.

"During the middle ages, the nations of Europe were periodically devastated by four distinct forms of plague-the plague proper, the sweating sickness, the black death and small pox. They were each about equally fatal and each most at home in squalor and filth. During the last century, in consequence of improved sanitation, three of the scourges have practically disappeared in the West, though they continue in the Orient where sanitary laws are quite unknown. In the West, we have only small pox left which should have departed with the other three, and would have departed had the doctors and the state brought to the altar the same disinterested solitude to secure general sanitation which they have displayed to enforce vaccination."[143] Instead of cleaning up the environment, they vaccinated instead. This is what we are doing now in third world countries.

Doctors claim that the science has been answered, but Bernadine Healy the former head of the National Institute of Health explained how there are some people who cannot be vaccinated which is a good reason not to mandate them but rather customize for each person. She said, "There is a completely expressed concern that they don't want to pursue a hypothesis because that hypothesis could be damaging to the public health community at large by scaring people. First of all, I think the public's smarter than that. The public values vaccines. But more importantly, I don't think you should ever turn your back on any scientific hypothesis because you're afraid of what it might show."[144]

People think that if you refuse vaccines you have not done the research but some of the smartest people have skipped or delayed vaccines. The daycare centers of six out of twelve technology company's home of Berkeley and Stanford are vaccinated at lower rates than average.[145] In other words, smart people do not vaccinate as much as everyone else because they have done the research.

What is the Link Between Vaccines and Autism?

Judy Mikovits, a Ph.D. in biochemistry and author of Plague said, "Vaccines do not cause autism. We cannot use the word cause or cure. The word cause is only used when every single case has a vaccine origin. What we usually say is associated. Are vaccines associated, do they play a role in brain damage, and immune system damage that results in autism? I would say absolutely and there is a ton of data to back that up."[146]

The circumstantial evidence is strong in some cases. There are studies in monkeys which show that they develop autism if they get the same vaccines at the same schedule that humans receive. Macaque monkeys vaccinated using the CDC schedule of the 1990s exhibited behavior changes similar to those displayed by children with autism.[147]

Dr. William Thompson revealed that he and his cohorts had covered up evidence that a study in 2004 found a 3.4 times increased risk of autism for African American males given the MMR vaccine before 36 months.[148] This is a long-complicated story and I will explain it in more detail in *Hiding the Liability and Risk of Vaccine Injuries*. You can also read the transcript when Thompson revealed his malfeasance and those of his cohorts in the book *Vaccine*

Whistleblower: Exposing Autism Research Fraud at the CDC, listed in Appendix O.

There are many doctors who have considered evidence against a link as circumstantial evidence and see that vaccines play a role in autism diagnosis. Dr. Mayer Eisenstein, who founded and was Medical Director of the Eisenstein Medical Centers who has cared for 50,000 children who were minimally or not vaccinated at all. He stated "There is virtually no autism, asthma, allergies, respiratory illness, or diabetes in these unvaccinated children, a telltale revelation when compared to national rates."[149]

This next case I share demonstrates that autism could have been avoided not by skipping the vaccine but changing when an injured person received it. I interviewed Linda Weinmaster on my radio show *Kitchen Sink Autism: Everything but the Kitchen Sink Related to Autism,* so she could tell her story about how the timing of the Rhogam shot changed with her third son, Adam, because the schedule for the CDC changed when he was born. She had the Rhogam shot for all three of her children but only one developed autism. In this case, Adam would have avoided getting an autism diagnosis if she had the shot after birth as she did with her other two sons.

Her whole ordeal could have been prevented if she had the shot after giving birth. The Rhogam shot is given during pregnancy for that child and for future children even though Linda would receive a tubal ligation. She said, "I had already signed the paper stating I wanted to have a tubal ligation when I had my third C-section. So, I wasn't going to have any future pregnancies so the shot was a waste."

Linda's doctor did not check for certain markers, alter the schedule or notice that there was anything wrong. Linda's sons and her husband played football and were very tall and muscular. The mercury in the Rhogam, the MTHFR gene, the testosterone in the family all lead to Adam's behavior regressing into autism and Linda's health suffered because of her Multiple Sclerosis. All of them could have been avoided by altering the schedule to get the shot after birth as she did with her first two sons, Phillip and Kyle, who do not have autism. You can listen to the whole interview on my website, breakingtheautismcode.com.

All this information confirms that the schedule can and should be altered, or changed to fit each person. Linda could have had the old vaccine schedule which did not keep her from getting the Rhogam shot just changed when it was given. If she had this shot as she did with her other two sons, perhaps her third child would not be on the spectrum.

Doctors: What Do They Know? What Don't They Know?

Doctors are taught that vaccines don't cause autism, and that is technically correct if you use the word cause. However, this is more about informed consent and circumstantial evidence. Has your doctor read the vaccine inserts? Has your doctor completed his own research and looked at circumstantial evidence between when these diseases started and when there was a vaccine? Do your legislators read the data? How about your school board?

Who has the right to decide your medical decisions or of your child? Do presidential candidates decide, your doctor, do you get to decide what gets injected into your own body? There is no one who does more research than a parent with a sick child. This is a moral right and it's a slippery slope where we have lost our own ability to take care of ourselves.

Informed consent is defined by the American Medical Association, which says that your doctor has a responsibility to "present the medical facts accurately to the patient or to the individual responsible for the patient's care and to make recommendations for management in accordance with good medical practice."[150]

Doctors ask you to read an information statement which does not give informed consent. It does not list all the side effects that the vaccine insert does. I have compared the two in Appendix J. Chances are, the doctor has not read the insert either. How would you feel if there was an information statement about thalidomide a drug used for morning sickness, that caused birth deformities? You would feel deceived if your child's deformity was called a coincidence. Should thalidomide be mandated? It has risks, and so do vaccines. Professionals mandate vaccines because they want to help humanity and save lives. If vaccines are mandated, anything, even thalidomide could be next.

What Are Vaccine Risks?

Doctors will tell you that we vaccine so often for herd immunity, yet some vaccines like tetanus do not spread person to person, and are not contagious.[151] The CDC claims that this vaccine is the most effective within three days before any signs of tetanus show up.

The incubation period of tetanus is 3-21 days. If you have tetanus, is it necessary to stay away from other children in school, since it is not contagious, and they cannot catch it? They can however catch pertussis which is in the same shot. Meaning the CDC wants you to get a vaccine before the disease shows up, claiming credit that the vaccine prevented a disease before it can manifest. Is it a coincidence when you do get tetanus after you were vaccinated, and the incubation period is over?

The risk of tetanus is increased if you live in a disaster area, or on a farm. The "outbreaks of tetanus were in places like tsunami sites."[152] Tetanus spores can be found in the intestines and feces of farm animals and in the soil.[153] Vaccines for tetanus are for personal protection only. Catholic Bishops raised an alarm in Kenya to refuse the tetanus vaccine for females because they say it caused infertility because it contains beta HCG.[154] There also happens to be a birth control injection that is coming out that happens to contain tetanus and is made from beta HCG.[155]

If there is a risk, there must be exemptions. The risks of vaccines are medical complications as well as mental ones. Also, people with autoimmunity like Lupus are more likely to have children on the spectrum than those without the disease.[156] Many of the people who skip, alter or delay vaccines, do so because they have vaccine injuries in the family besides autism.

Vaccines are associated with encephalitis, autoimmunity, and anaphylactic shock to name a few. These are serious and life threatening for some individuals. We cannot mandate any medication that can cause that great of a risk.

The Merck Manual states the following as the definition. "Encephalitis is inflammation of the brain that occurs when a virus directly infects the brain or when a virus, vaccine or something else triggers inflammation. The spinal cord may also be involved, resulting in a disorder called encephalomyelitis."[157]

Encephalitis is linked to mental disorders such as motor impairment, mental retardation, epilepsy, ADHD, and learning disorders.[158] All of these are often present at the same time as autistic behaviors.

Encephalitis is a type of autoimmunity. Vaccines are linked to autoimmune diseases where the immune system attacks itself. Autoimmunity covers a wide range of disorders. It plays a role in autism,[159] Lupus, MS, ALS, and Rheumatoid Arthritis.[160] Autoimmunity is linked to vaccines and many other things. ASIA meaning Autoimmune Inflammatory Syndrome is linked to some of the vaccine ingredients.[161]

The Centers for Disease Control indicates that the Hepatitis B vaccine is not linked to Multiple Sclerosis, but a French study showed a correlation between Hepatitis B and MS that is causal.[162]

Anaphylaxis is a severe allergy and is listed on several vaccine inserts according to Health and Human Services. The following vaccines list it as a side effect including Varicella, Influenza, Hepatitis B, Meningococcal, MMR and DPT.[163] The CDC again says that this risk is minor.[164] You have the right to know about this adverse event, if it does happen and the doctors should be better informed so you can do something about it.

Another risk that is often discussed on television is a risk of gastrointestinal disorders. An example of such a study is one by Karolyn Horvath, MD, and her colleagues, who state that "unrecognized gastrointestinal disorders, especially reflux esophagitis and disaccharide mal-absorption, may contribute to the behavioral problems of the non-verbal autistic patients."[165]

Vaccine Ingredients: Which Offer the Greatest Risks?

Vaccines contain Aluminum, Thimerosal, aborted fetal tissue, polysorbate 80, and nagalase, all of which sometimes in combination are risks to vulnerable populations. An investigation of vaccines begins not just in each ingredient, but with each other or with other inert environmental components. These ingredients become dangerous because they bypass the body's natural defenses, damage the defenses in the gut, and stay in the body longer than anticipated. The gut the brain and the immune system work together and it matters greatly that these are injected which bypasses the gut to go further in the body.

Aluminum

Aluminum by itself can result in brain and immune issues especially in premature babies. We cannot compare eating and drinking aluminum with direct injection. Health and Human Services argues that aluminum in food water and medicine leave the body quickly in the feces. The small amount that does enter the bloodstream leaves quickly through the urine.[166] Aluminum, however, injected via a vaccine, stays in the body causing brain and immune issues.[167] The total load from vaccines that babies receive is up to 4,925 mcg by 18 months of age.[168] The FDA says that

25 mcg is safe per day.[169] The Hepatitis B Vaccine contains 250 mcg by itself.[170]

"Children from countries with the highest ASD prevalence appear to have the highest exposure to Aluminum from vaccines. Also, the increase in exposure to Aluminum adjuvant significantly correlates with the increase in Autism prevalence in the United States, observed over the last two decades. A significant correlation exists between the amounts of aluminum administered to preschool children and the current prevalence of ASD in seven Western countries, particularly at 3-4 months of age,"[171] per Dr. Christopher Shaw.

The population at risk from aluminum are premature babies, the elderly and those with poor kidney function. Babies who are exposed to aluminum may have reduced lumbar spine and hipbone mass during adolescence, potential risk factors for later osteoporosis and hip fracture.[172] This means that if the aluminum accumulated in the bones of the baby, he might be weaker and more prone to fractures. Aluminum crosses the blood brain barrier and affects ALS, Parkinson's, and dementia. Shaken baby syndrome diagnosed with swelling of the brain, bleeding of the surface of the brain and back of the eyes can have other reasons than a baby being shaken.[173] Child Abuse symptoms are like the symptoms of infantile rickets.[174] Osteocalcin, or soft bones, can also be associated with aluminum.[175] Injected aluminum hydroxide stays in the body, and accumulates in the kidney to impair kidney function.[176]

When someone is exposed to both aluminum and peanut oil at the same time, the immune system fights the peanut oil the same way it would fight an infection. Peanut oil is a vaccine ingredient but this can also happen to a child who eats peanuts around the time the injection of aluminum is given. In the movie, *Age of Aluminum*, filmmakers demonstrate that when testing peanut allergy medications, they create the allergy first in the rats, and they do this by injecting aluminum followed by peanut oil.[177]

Mercury

The Centers for Disease Control considers that mercury is safe in vaccines because it leaves the body quickly. It was removed years ago, as a precaution, and the amount left in vaccines is only considered to be trace amounts. This is deceptive because mercury is toxic even down to minute levels, and mercury is still in multi dose injected flu shots. This mercury combined with ingredients in other vaccines are much more toxic than either one alone, and quite damaging to pregnant women.

A study in 2002 studied thimerosal measuring mercury in the blood, stool and urine. This study concluded that the ethyl mercury would be eliminated from the body rapidly because he could not find it in the blood, saliva or hair.[178] However, another study found that the mercury did in fact leave the blood quickly and went straight to the brain.[179]

Safeminds found that autism and mercury poisoning were associated because the symptoms of mercury poisoning and of autism are virtually identical.[180] Robert Kennedy Junior has been studying the effects of thimerosal for many years, and commented in his speech at the Autism One Conference in 2013. "Thimerosal causes autism in sheep, monkeys, goats, and dogs, but it's fine for humans. That's what they told us."[181] Mercury is not just toxic by itself though; it's much more toxic when combined with other ingredients.

The combination of vaccine ingredients or when these ingredients are combined with other environmental sources of toxicity are deadly. Mercury combined with aluminum, lead or arsenic are also toxic. In this study the amounts of thimerosal killed 1 in 100 rats, and the amount of aluminum killed 1 in 100 rats but aluminum and thimerosal together killed 100% of the rats.[182] If you combine the flu shot with another vaccine on the schedule that contains aluminum at the same visit, it's much more toxic, or if the child already has the mercury in his body.

The Centers for Disease Control said in July 1999, "that thimerosal should be reduced or eliminated in vaccines as a precautionary measure." [183] However, it was still included in multi dose vials of flu shots. These shots are given to pregnant women and the elderly. The Full Prescribing Information for Flulaval indicates that safety and effectiveness has not been established for pregnant women and antibody responses were lower in the geriatric population.[184] Eli Lilly, the manufacturer of thimerosal, says on their safety data sheet that mercury in utero causes mild to severe mental retardation and mild to severe motor coordination. It also lists liver, lung, kidney and nervous system problems.[185]

Other Important Vaccine Ingredients

Vaccines also contain other ingredients made from aborted fetal cells, animal DNA, and nagalase. The aborted fetal cells are listed as MRC-5 and WI38. Vaccines for Hepatitis A, German Measles, chicken pox and rabies contain these cells. Dr. Paul Offit admitted that vaccines contain aborted fetal cells when he said, "German Measles, also known as rubella caused 5000 abortions a year. We wouldn't have saved all those lives, if it weren't for those cells."[186]

Some other important ingredients include formaldehyde, bovine extract, monkey kidney tissue, DNA, insect egg protein, egg protein, chicken kidney cells, calf serum protein, monkey kidney tissue, chicken protein, and fetal bovine serum.[187] Polysorbate 80 is an ingredient in vaccines that causes infertility in rats.[188]

According to the late Jeffery Bradstreet MD vaccines also contain nagalase, a vitamin D binding protein found in vaccines, leading to immune suppression in cancer patients. [189,190] In other words, some people cannot be vaccinated because of immune suppression, and this ingredient causes immune suppression.

Aluminum, mercury and other ingredients in vaccines are linked to autoimmunity, allergies and immune suppression and some of these ingredients when combined or alone are associated with autism in some cases. If we take away just one ingredient, it won't diminish autism completely because the problem is the entire schedule with all the ingredients together, the timing of the vaccine to the timing of the disease, and that the vaccines are not tested to properly and not guaranteed to work.

Who is Vulnerable to Vaccine Injury?

The most vulnerable people who should not be vaccinated are those with a history of vaccine injuries.

The Young Family

The first question to ask as to who should not be vaccinated is to inquire if there is vaccine injury in the family, because often this is multigenerational and as this example shows there are different reactions to different vaccines. I am adding Maria's letter in its entirety here because it's important to see her story along with a family history of people who cannot handle the toxicity and ingredients in vaccines. I have included her story as well because her mother, father, grandfather, brother and uncle were all injured by vaccines in a different way, and because her mother, father and her grandfather were medical professionals who know and understand how vaccines work.

Because of these subsequent injuries, Maria's father, Clay Young, MD, no longer offers vaccines to his patients. Now her family is part of a much larger group working to educate others about vaccine injuries. Marie's parents, Virginia and Clay have the scientific background to validate these injuries. Both of Maria's parents are graduates of A&M University and both have a Bachelor of Science degree in biomedical science. They both worked in research in the Texas Medical Center. They then returned to College Station. Clay graduated from Texas A&M University Health Science Center College of Medicine while Virginia completed her Master of Science degree in Kinesiology with emphasis in Exercise Physiology.

Clay completed his residency in Obstetrics and Gynecology at Scott and White Memorial Hospital and Clinic in 1998. While her husband was in residency, Virginia worked as a fitness instructor, personal trainer, and in-home child care giver. She sat on the Board of the American Heart Association of Bell County, chaired two American Heart Walks, and volunteered extensively for organizations such as the Children's Miracle Network, Juvenile Diabetes Foundation, and March of Dimes. Marie's grandfather was once President of the AMA in Texas.

Maria was not the first in her family to have a vaccine injury but she was the last straw in a group who were vaccine injured. Her struggles were the beginning of her family's research to find out whether vaccines were worth the risk. Marie's uncle recently passed in May of 2013 after receiving the flu vaccine in the hospital. He had been admitted to the critical care unit for a grand mal seizure of unknown origin and while there he was given the flu vaccine. He died from blunt force trauma to his head from a fall in the hospital before he recovered. His sister, Virginia believed the post vaccine reaction which left him debilitated precipitated the event and could most definitely have been prevented.

Maria's father received the Hepatitis B vaccine in medical school. He was told he must do so to continue his studies. His subsequent leg pain, migraine headaches, and memory loss left him bed ridden for days. Her mother was hospitalized with an illness of unknown origin affecting her urinary tract system. Surgery gave no clues. The illness hit at ages 5, 11, and later at 18. By the age of 18 she realized the doctors did not have any answers nor did they have any treatments. She had been told that she would most likely "outgrow the symptoms" as she had done earlier. Similar symptoms appeared in her 20s as well as a possible cardiac arrhythmia and other neurological and respiratory symptoms that would come and go without explanation. These same symptoms reappeared after an event at the age of 33. This time she would experience an assault on her whole body within minutes of a tetanus shot. She nearly lost control of her car as she drove home from the emergency room.

Unfortunately, when we vaccinate by force, medical professionals are often the first to be vaccinated, and the Young family have all suffered subsequent vaccine injuries, and therefore they refuse vaccines for themselves or for their patients. Virginia Young, Maria's mother is an advocate for vaccine injured families and I am honored she would share the family's stories with me.

This is the letter Maria wrote about herself and her twin brother, as testimony about what happens to Vaccine Injured Victims:

> "We were born a little early in 1997, at 34 weeks and 4 days and at just under 5 pounds each, but we were amazingly healthy. The nurses and doctors all remarked at how healthy and strong we were. We were dismissed from the NICU in 24 hours, and although we were small we were given the Hepatitis B vaccine at 10 days of age. At that point in time we were still premature and barely 36 weeks old. The next day I was covered in the rash you see still on my body today. The rash was far worse than it is today, but it would subside only to return always and only after shots. The doctors still would say that shots wouldn't cause it but they also say they don't know what causes my illness known as Urticaria Pigmentosa."

> "My brother and I reacted to each and every one of our shots. Our fevers would shoot up to 106 or 107 degrees sometimes. In some cases, we were covered in rashes and hives. At one time, we were left unable to walk and what words we had learned were lost. We were injected at the same time and fell violently ill at the same time. When we were one-year-old it was at 1:10 am and she said her skin burned to hold us. There is a good chance we had seizures, but all was ignored.

The only word I would or could say was 'cupcake.' I would start learning everything from name and age and all had I had learned to that point all over again. I was three at the time and the shot was Medimmune. I have struggled to learn ever since, but with hindsight we know this was not the only reaction that I suffered and I was not the only one to react."

The Young family, full of medical professionals, have all been injured from vaccines refuse them because they do not want what happened to them to happen to anyone else. That's the same reason I write this book and the same reason parents want choice in what is injected into their children or into themselves. Unfortunately, the only way some doctors seem to understand this is when they themselves are injured. It takes a brave soul, especially a doctor, to stand up against vaccines because there is a severe push back from the medical community. Virginia and her family are brave, and I hope that if you are injured, you will be brave too.

Lisa Mark Smith

Lisa Mark Smith's story was different than Maria Young's story because there was no history of vaccine injuries and no sign that there would be any reason why she should not get a flu shot. She was a healthy normal weight forty-two-year-old who walked four miles a day and was basically barely ever sick. Lisa had decided to get her flu shot, Fluzone, which was offered at her local drug store. Lisa's father had just had knee surgery and Lisa spent a lot of time with him in the hospital.

I have included her story because she is someone whose only clue that she could be injured was eczema. Her doctors did not understand it was the flu shot because some doctors are not informed of the risk. If she had not gone to a better hospital she might have died.

In 1958, it was already clear that children with eczema should not be vaccinated. No family member of those with eczema should be vaccinated either.[191] Yet, Lisa was still vaccinated. We have since changed this rule but in her case, it could have saved her.

I have also included her story because some behaviors she had such as OCD, fatigue, walking on her toes, short term memory loss, and her skin felt inflamed and too painful to be touched are sometimes seen in children on the spectrum, but her case was not autism but caused by the flu shot, and an autism parent will see similarities. The court said she had "Post Infectious Myositis due to the flu vaccine." She had muscle and nerve damage with known lead, mercury, and cadmium in her blood. Her story is showing that her flu shot changed her personality, her memory and the way her body functioned.

Lisa began to feel sick a day or two after the shot. She says "It's weird I have a little tickle in my throat." The next day, I woke up just full-blown sick. I had a fever like 103, felt awful. Then my husband, we called the doctor. Of course, they weren't in on the weekend and they said they could get me in on Monday. By Monday, I just said to him, "I think I need to go to the emergency room because I feel like I am going to die."

Soon, Lisa could no longer walk down the stairs. She went to the emergency room and the doctors told her she had pneumonia and put her on antibiotics. That did not fix her situation because at this point, Lisa could barely walk or move at all and she was becoming worse. Two weeks later, Lisa went in an ambulance to the hospital. She could only move her head at this point and she had "foot drop" where her feet would hang loose. Doctors didn't test her and said her symptoms were psychogenic or, in other words, she was making it up. Lisa and her family became fed up with the lack of care and attention at this hospital and transferred her to another better one.

The doctors at the second hospital realized from a blood test that confirmed that something was causing the protein levels in her blood to go down and her muscles were decaying. Her nerves were damaged as well.

"You could not touch me because the nerve endings were so inflamed. Kind of like a burn patient, like if you touch me I would just scream because the pain was so bad. But I could not use the muscles in my legs at all. I mean I could not sit up."

Lisa noticed other problems like a short-term memory loss, sound sensitivity, sensory overload, and poor word recall. Her speech became very blunt where she would insert words into a conversation that made no sense. The word chair would be added into a sentence, because she was looking at a chair. She also began to have obsessive-compulsive behavior, buying an endless supply of v-neck shirts. She also began to walk on her toes and could not put her heels down. Lisa nicknamed this "Barbie feet".

Doctors were at a loss as to what they could do for Lisa and basically told her she was going to die because there was nothing else they could do for her. They told her to get her affairs in order and say goodbye to her family. One doctor, her neurologist did not lose hope. She told Lisa to see a chiropractor, or try acupuncture or just try anything to heal.

Later doctors confirmed that Lisa had peroneal neuropathy or nerve damage in her feet. The actual medical diagnosis was "Post Infectious Myositis due to the flu vaccine." Myositis means muscle damage. She also had some myelitis, nerve damage, but the doctor said there was more muscle then nerve damage. She also had high levels of Mercury, Cadmium and Lead in her blood. One doctor told her the high levels of mercury were from eating too much seafood. Lisa didn't eat seafood.

It is very difficult to find any accountability in Lisa's situation. By law, Lisa could not sue the doctor, the hospital or the pharmacy where she had her flu vaccine. She took her case to "vaccine court" and won her case. Even though the flu shot almost killed her, Lisa is alive and can walk now because she took her doctor's advice and found a Naturopath to remove the metals from her body and help her heal the damage in her legs and feet. Lisa still has some issues but she can walk now without the wheelchair.

Lisa is testimony of the harm that a flu shot can cause in a healthy individual. She learned later that she was at risk to vaccine injury because she had eczema. Lisa's advocacy extended to her son's school because she did not want her son to get the same flu shot that nearly killed her and that school still couldn't understand why even after seeing her in a wheel chair earlier.

What Do I Need to Know about Limited Immunity from Vaccines?

Some studies indicate that certain vaccines spread diseases instead of offer protection. The Flumist and the Acellular Pertussis portion of the DTAP are two such examples. These studies are showing that the vaccinated are giving the disease to others even without symptoms.

The Flumist is a vaccine that can spread the flu to others through "shedding." The Highlights of Prescribing Information for Flumist claims it is to "prevent influenza not cause it" yet it also states that "viral shedding is necessary for the vaccine to work," and that people who get vaccinated have symptoms such as runny nose, nasal congestion and sore throat, and fever for up to 28 days with symptoms similar to the flu.[192,193]

The Flumist vaccine insert says that between 1-7% were shedding the live virus through nasal secretions for up to 28 days' post vaccination.[194] This is not listed in the vaccine information statements given to parents at the time the vaccine is given.

Pertussis can also spread to others even if you have been vaccinated without showing symptoms. A study in 2014 concluded that the baboons who were given the acellular pertussis portion of the DTAP vaccine and later exposed may have no further symptoms of pertussis but were still transmitting it other unvaccinated baboons. "Baboons were vaccinated at two, four and six months of age with aP or whole cell pertussis and though they were protected from severe symptoms of pertussis, they were still readily transmitting it to unvaccinated contacts.[195] What does this mean? It means that these baboons, even if they had no symptoms of pertussis, were still spreading disease. This means that the vaccinated were spreading pertussis not the unvaccinated.

The CDC says "Many babies and young children get whooping cough from adults or older brothers or sisters who don't know they have the disease. Pregnant women with whooping cough can give it to their newborn babies. Because whooping cough is so harmful in babies, everyone around them needs to be up-to-date with vaccines - to make a circle of protection." [196] We are in fact spreading pertussis to our babies when we create that "circle of protection" because we are spreading pertussis when we get a vaccine even without symptoms.

What is the Connection Between Autism at Birth and Vaccine Injury?

There is a great contradiction in the fact that the CDC continues to tell pregnant mothers to get vaccines, yet in some cases the vaccine insert says that the vaccine has not been tested on pregnant women.

In another study with mice, the risk of autism occurs when the mother has been exposed to a virus while pregnant.[197] This is what happens when you inject a vaccine. In mice, this single insult to the mother translates into autism-related behavioral abnormalities and neuropathology in the offspring.

How Do I Get the Facts to Make an Informed Decision?

When you go to the doctor, he hands you a piece of paper called a Vaccine Information Statement, which will tell you all the risks, because it comes from the CDC. If everyone read the vaccine insert they may consider that risk more carefully. Isn't it important to know all the risks just like you would any other medication?

An example of the difference between the Vaccine Information Statement you receive from your doctor at the time of vaccination and the vaccine insert is that the vaccine insert offers more details. For example, the insert for Infanrix says that it has not been evaluated for fertility, carcinogenic or mutagenic potential.[198] That means a doctor can truthfully say that there are no studies that conclude that vaccines cause cancer because there are no studies done to check at all.

The Vaccine Information Statement is not as comprehensive as the vaccine insert which makes it difficult for parents to have an informed decision at well child visits. Even if these issues are rare it is important for the patients as well as doctors to know about them and acknowledge that they can and do occur or they would not be listed in the vaccine insert.

The stories listed in this book are parents who had reactions such as this should not be dismissed, or put down or labeled as a coincidence if the child develops an injury that is clearly stated in the vaccine insert. If it appears in the vaccine insert but not in the vaccine information statement it should at the very least be investigated thoroughly.

I wrote this not just for parents of kids on the spectrum but to explain to the general population that they may be injured from a vaccine and not be aware. If they suspect that they were injured or their child changed after a vaccine, then it's time to investigate the data and seek further input. It's time for everyone who has had a vaccine injury to stand as one group and demand some accountability from the court system, the pharmaceutical companies and the CDC and FDA to allow that there are some people with a lower immunity or have a family history of vaccine damage who should not be vaccinated and there are others who should delay certain vaccines. This is a danger to no one but the child who receives the vaccine.

Downplaying the Risk:
Hiding the Liability and Risk of Vaccine Injuries

One way to prevent or minimize autistic like symptoms is to avoid vaccines. This remedy is controversial, but I will argue that it is one of the most important steps we can take as parents. If your children have already been vaccine injured, it's important to avoid or minimize future vaccines and thus avoiding future injuries especially with injuries in other family members. If you have children with vaccine injuries, I'll be able to offer some friendly advice to prevent further damage. But first, I want to share the latest research on vaccine injury, and explain the incentive to hide the dangers of current vaccines and vaccination schedules.

We have been taught to believe that vaccines will always work, and that the medical community always has the consumer's best interest to make us healthy. We have faith that they never lie, cheat, or make a mistake. Hillary Clinton said in a tweet, "The science is clear, the earth is round, the sky is blue, and vaccines work."[199] But consumers need to think like scientists to understand the problem we face with vaccine development and distribution.

True science is investigation and peer review, not blind faith that leads us to treat our doctor like a God, listening to his sermon about vaccine safety, and ignoring injuries we can see with our own eyes. We also need to pay attention to the power behind the doctors, and the reasons pharmaceutical companies want us to believe their products are safe. There is a whole industry built up to protect vaccines with propaganda.

Profit is the route and reason for all the corruption in the vaccine industry. There is malfeasance, deception and corruption from the financial ties of the scientists to their protocols of ethics, health, and safety. We are dependent on medications and vaccines for life, but the industry maintains a balance that makes sure we are just healthy enough to need them for life but not sick enough to die. Pharmaceutical companies will keep offering us medications and vaccines if we keep asking for them, even when they wear off or do not work at all. If they cause more symptoms, we take more pills and more shots to fix those. We are dependent on medications and vaccines to stay alive, but too sick to research if the same medications are causing the problem in the first place. Bill Maher put it perfectly, "There is no money in dead people, and there is no money in healthy people. The money is the middle. The people who are alive--sort of -- but with one or more chronic conditions."[200]

Scientists are financially dependent on the companies whose products they are supposed to be testing for safety. Congressman Dan Burton criticized this practice:

"The CDC routinely allows scientists with blatant conflicts of interest to serve on influential advisory committees that make recommendations on new vaccines, while these same scientists have financial ties, academic affiliations and other vested interests in the products and companies for which they are supposed to be providing unbiased oversight."[201]

We did not know until recently how many mistakes or how many studies have been manipulated to profit from a sick and tired population. The Centers for Disease Control (CDC), founded in 1946, was more appropriately known as the Communicable Disease Center until 1992.[202] Their data and scientists are considered the gold standard for integrity of not just vaccines, but all medications. But this belief is dangerous. When we learn the truth, we believe nothing that they do or say. We should also mistrust the FDA, our doctors and the pharmaceutical companies because the same scientists are manipulating the science in both the government and the private sector and making themselves rich as we become sick and tired, medically and emotionally.

The ethics and morals of companies and government agencies that are supposed to be protecting the public are called into question when they promote drugs that are not safe like Vioxx, or don't follow safety protocols because the CDC, FDA and NIH were careless leaving deadly diseases lying around in a box. Sometimes foundations such as Bill and Melinda Gates foundation have tested a vaccine such as Gardasil and Cervarix on unsuspecting illiterate girls who have no informed consent.

Sometimes drug companies pay heavy fines for promotion of products that they know cause harm. Pfizer paid 2.3 billion dollars for an illegal marketing scheme of promoting Bextra for "post-operative pain" even though it was not approved for that use.[203] Merck paid $950 million for promoting Vioxx when it increased risk for heart attacks. Glaxo Smith Kline paid a fine of 3 billion to promote Paxil for people under 18 when it was not approved for that age group. Johnson and Johnson paid 3 billion to push Risperdal for psychotic symptoms for non-schizophrenic patients when it was only approved for schizophrenia.[204] Risperdal is sometimes used as a medication for autism.

But vaccine manufacturers rarely pay any fines if the vaccines are defective because there is no accountability built into vaccine regulation. The Bill and Melinda Gates Foundation were testing the Gardasil and Cervix vaccines on poor and illiterate girls who had no informed consent and suffered injuries and even death in some cases in India in 2009. Seven girls died with the cause of death listed as "suicide, accidental drowning in well, malaria, viral infections, subarachnoid hemorrhage." 127 girls suffered injuries in what the India Supreme court called more of a drug trial than a study. 120 girls suffered with epileptic seizures, severe stomachache, headaches and mood swings, early menstruation, heavy bleeding, and menstrual cramps.[205]

There have been other dangerous trends in experiments with diseases. The CDC, FDA and NIH were also careless leaving deadly pathogens in a box which could have had disastrous consequences or even spread these diseases into the public domain. The United States regulators investigated to find 12 boxes of 327 vials labeled dengue, influenza, Q fever, and rickettsia as well as an earlier box of smallpox.[206]

There are consequences to the public if the manufacturers are less than honest about effectiveness of vaccines. The public blames the unvaccinated even if all the people who are sick have had their vaccines. The blame belongs with the manufacturers who have no accountability in the current system and have created inferior products. Merck allegedly misrepresented the truth because they were not honest about the efficacy of the Mumps portion of the MMR. There were two lawsuits about the efficacy of the mumps portion of the MMR vaccine to keep away competitors.[207] There was a recent mumps outbreak at Harvard University, yet all the students were vaccinated. Consider this lawsuit before you accept another dose of the MMR which didn't work twice already.[208]

The AIDS vaccines and the Lymerix vaccine for Lyme were heavily promoted as a cure but were not, in fact, effective. Dong-Pyou Han, a former Iowa State University Scientist also was indicted for faking lab results of the AIDS vaccine to obtain grant money because he had spiked rabbit blood with human antibodies.[209] Han was sentenced to 57 months in prison, plus required to pay $7,216,890.12 to the National Institute of Health.[210] Han's findings were reported in journals and he managed to receive 19 million in research grants, but his peers could not duplicate his results.[211] Lastly, Lymerix had a class action lawsuit because 121 people experienced arthritis or symptoms similar to Lyme, the disease it was intended to prevent. Lymerix was soon taken off the market for poor sales.[212,213]

Dr. Poul Thorsen, a scientist indicted for thirteen counts of fraud, wrote the most cited studies that prove there is no link between vaccines and autism. Thorsen is listed in the Office of Inspector General, as a fugitive.[214] He is currently missing and last seen in Denmark with his girlfriend Diane Schendel who used to work at the CDC, but now works at the Aarhus University, where they are still producing scholarly articles.[215]

He is the key source the CDC relies on for data. He has been indicted for money laundering because he stole two million dollars in grants from the CDC that should have been used for research. Thorsen, who coauthored 90 scientific papers and book chapters, says that when you take thimerosal, an ingredient identified with autistic-like symptoms, out of vaccines, the rates of autism go down.[216] However, he was only able to make this argument by changing the autism diagnosis which would exclude 75% of those with higher functioning vaccine injury symptoms.[217,218] This way the rates of autism go down because they reconfigured the criteria.

The MMR vaccine which does not contain mercury is still associated with autism. When parents have complained that their child regressed into autism after being given the MMR vaccine, there is proof directly from the CDC that this can and does happen. Congress needs to subpoena Dr. William Thompson to seek the truth in the matter. Dr. Thompson and his colleagues, Coleen Boyle, Frank Estefan, Tanya Bhasin, Marshalyn Yeargin-Allsopp, have not just hidden the data for over ten years, but literally threw it away for fear of discovery. The CDC has not studied autism in the past ten years afraid of what they might find.

Dr. Brian Hooker, PhD a scientist at Simpson University, and the father of a vaccine-injured child, began his research with Freedom of Information Act Requests to analyze the data the CDC uses to show no association between vaccines and autism.

Dr. Hooker legally recorded conversations with Dr. William Thompson who still works at the CDC. These conversations reveal that there is a positive link between the MMR vaccine and autism for young African American boys. They also explain that there were people who developed autism with no previous disability, and questioned why you ever give thimerosal to a pregnant woman.

As a scientist, certain rules must be followed to have complete and accurate data. This case reveals that the solution to the scientific experiment was altered to create a desired outcome. This not just corruption and fraud, but this faulty science harmed millions of children and that could have been avoided if they had told the truth.

Thompson explains how this fraud was carried out when he stated "All the authors and I met and decided sometime between August and September '02 not to report any trace effects from the paper. Sometime soon after the meeting we decided to exclude reporting any trace effects, the coauthors scheduled a meeting to destroy documents related to the study. The remaining four coauthors all met and brought a big garbage can into the meeting room and reviewed and went through all the hard-copy documents that we had thought we should discard and put them in a huge garbage can. However, because I assumed it was illegal and would violate both FOIA and Department of Justice requests, I kept hard copies of all documents in my office and I retained all associated computer files. I believe we intentionally withheld controversial findings from the final draft of the Pediatrics paper."[219]

People naturally would skip or delay at least some vaccines if they knew there was a problem with vaccines, but if the CDC and researchers were honest about the risks, perhaps we would not abandon the program completely. The CDC's lack of honesty did not create trust in the industry.

Thompson admits that he neglected some significant information that would help families decide which vaccines to get and when. Thompson said, "I regret that my coauthors and I omitted statistically significant information in our 2004 article published in the Journal of Pediatrics. The omitted data suggested that African American males who received the MMR vaccine before age 36 months were at increased risk for autism. Decisions were made regarding which findings to report after the data were collected, and I believe that the final study protocol was not followed."[220] When Dr. Brian Hooker reanalyzed the data in the 2004 study and found a "236% increase in risk of autism for African American males given MMR before aged 36 months."[221]

The CDC will not analyze anything even remotely connected to autism or it's symptoms. Thompson said, "We've missed ten years of research because the CDC is so paralyzed right now by anything related to autism. They're not doing what they should be doing because they're afraid to look for things that might be associated."[222]

Thompson's confession also proved that autism effected a population known as "isolated autism." These are kids with no family history of autism and no co-morbid disorder like cerebral palsy, mental retardation, visual impairment, hearing impairment, epilepsy or birth defects. Those with these conditions were called non-isolated autism.[223] This means that anyone, African American or not, is vulnerable to vaccine injuries.

Further the book analyzes thimerosal, the mercury in some flu shots to be associated with autism. He explained that vaccines are associated with tics if given during pregnancy. Tics are rapid sudden vocal or motor movements like twitching or blinking which happens at the same time as other disorders like ADHD or OCD.[224]

Thompson said "I can say confidently; I do think thimerosal causes tics. So, I don't know why they still give it to pregnant women. I would never give my wife a vaccine that I thought caused tics. I can say, tics are four times more prevalent in kids with autism. There is biologic plausibility right now to say that thimerosal causes autism-like symptoms."[225]

Thompson has forwarded thousands of documents to Congressman Bill Posey, a Republican from Florida to illuminate these new findings. Robert Kennedy Jr. has read these documents and said in a public statement: "This is not just a smoking gun but a wildfire that would burn the CDC down to its foundations."

The Thompson confessions were recorded by Dr. Brian Hooker, Ph.D. and you can read about it further in the 2015 book called *Vaccine Whistleblower,* by Kevin Barry. You also see more information in a documentary film, *Vaxxed: from Cover Up to Catastrophe,* currently traveling through the United States.

Dr. William Thompson has given Congressman Posey 10,000 documents that will show Congress that the CDC has allegedly lied about vaccines and the connection to autism for over a decade. Congressman Posey has spoken in front of Congress twice to get Thompson's confessions in public record and to request that a hearing convene to subpoena Thompson to reveal all the data to the public. With revelations like this, the CDC now seems more like the Wizard of Oz hiding behind the curtain pulling the strings to make them seem more great and powerful than they really are. Posey does not have the authority to bring this case forward, but has requested that Congressman Jason Chaffetz do so. He has not.

If they had had told the truth from the very beginning, so much damage would be prevented. Yet the CDC has consistently stated that there is no link between the MMR vaccine and autism and no link between thimerosal an ingredient in multi dose flu shots. Thompson's testimony puts the entire fabric of the FDA, CDC and pharmaceutical companies as well as our doctors under high scrutiny if we are told the truth.

Many people who benefit from the profits of vaccines happen to also decide if these same vaccines are put on to the CDC vaccine schedule. For example, Julie Gerberding, Thompson's boss, and the CDC former director, and Dr. Paul Offit of the Children's Hospital of Philadelphia, both profited from distributed vaccines. Ms. Gerberding made a handsome profit from the MMR vaccine, while Paul Offit made a nice profit from RotaTeq.

Julie Gerberding sold 38,369 shares of Merck for 2.3 million dollars.[226] She was once the Director of the Centers for Disease Control and has since moved to the head of the vaccine division at Merck, the maker of the MMR vaccine.

She uses the Institute of Medicine as validation that the MMR vaccine is safe, but also is a member. That's basically like saying, "The MMR is safe because I say so." She is in both groups so she can use her own studies to prove vaccines are safe.

She said, "There have been at least 15 very good scientific studies on the Institute of Medicine who have searched this out. And they have concluded that there really is no association between vaccines and autism."[227] For someone who is going to move over to work for Merck, she had better tow the company line.

Paul Offit invented and patented the RotaTeq vaccine, while on the committee that decides to put it on the schedule. Should the inventor of a vaccine get to decide to put his own vaccine on the CDC schedule? This invention was "like winning the lottery," he said.[228] Offit was doctor at the Children's Hospital of Philadelphia and a member of the US Advisory Committee of Immunization Practices.[229]

Andrew Wakefield had his career ruined by writing one paper[230] sharing research that found gastrointestinal complaints and developmental delays in children linked to the MMR vaccine. This is Brian Hooker's list of 28 papers that prove Dr. Wakefield's hypothesis was correct; I list them here in the back of this book[231] in Appendix K.

For 13 years, the General Medical Council in the UK prosecuted Wakefield, John Walker-Smith and Dr. Murch which resulted in their medical licenses being revoked for the paper they published in 1998 that found gastrointestinal damage in 12 children after receiving the MMR vaccine. The paper concluded that the MMR vaccine should be split into three separate vaccines. It never stated that vaccines cause autism but that further study was needed.[232]

Ten of his coauthors signed a paper that vaccines do not cause autism which the paper did not prove. Andrew Wakefield, John Walker Smith, and Simon Murch were charged by the General Medical council of medical misconduct, but Simon Murch never lost his medical license. Dr. Walker-Smith regained his medical license after 14 years and his medical license was restored. Justice John Mitting said in the Walker-Smith appeal about the original trial, The GMC trial had "inadequate and superficial reasoning and, in a number of instances, a wrong conclusion."[233,234]

If the science is faked, and scientists make money from your child's illness, then it is not science but greed. Yet if true science shows what is contrary to popular beliefs, why do we still trust the CDC and other organizations? Why do we believe that the science has been asked and answered?

Please review the vaccine inserts before getting a vaccine and know what is injected. We cannot just blindly get a vaccine when it is not tested for safety, or it does not work as intended. We as individual families decide what is best for our families. Please write to Jason Chaffetz and to your own congressman to bring this hearing forward and receive justice for the kids who are injured.

Part 5: Friendly Advice on Detoxification, Diets and IEP Success

How to Change Your Family Diet and Support Detoxification?

Universal Rules of Diets

- Don't try every diet at once. This can seem quite overwhelming and these diets may not all be necessary for everyone.
- A Herxheimer Reaction[235] means you get worse before you get better. Sometimes kids get a "die off" reaction meaning though the behaviors may get worse from a few days to a few weeks, the body is in a state of healing but it takes time.
- Don't beat yourself up. Everyone occasionally forgets or slips and eats these foods. There are so many celebrations that it's heartbreaking not to give your child these foods even when you know the behaviors and diarrhea that may result.
- If you do give your child a food and he has a bad reaction, you can give him activated charcoal which will absorb what is in the gut and remove it. This will also remove medications so take it away from when your child takes them. It is also useful to have with any sort of stomach upset.

- Move forward one meal at time and one diet at a time. Figure out what your child will eat for seven days just breakfast, then dinner, then lunch and snack. You may have to play with the menu that both satisfies the diet and what your child will eat.
- Try juicing and smoothies to get kids to eat the fruit and veggies. Kids may eat the veggies if they can't taste them so easily. Mixing in vegetables that are the same color of the food you are eating can sneak in some nutrition.
- Celebrate small victories such as spoon of this or a bite of that. Sometimes that's enough.
- Taper the addicting foods slowly. A smoothie with real milk then half real milk and half almond milk until the real milk is gone. These foods are addicting, and your child may miss the "high" from eating those foods.
- Kids chronically constipated need a regular clean out.

Three Ways To Clean the Gut

I recommend non-pill related relief for long-term use, since prescription laxatives are only recommended for short-term use.[236]

Vitamin C Cleanse. [237] Vitamin C helps clear out of impacted fecal matter that has built up in the intestines. Your child may need a periodic cleanout to make sure the digestive system is working to its full potential. Be sure to use buffered ascorbic acid. The basic directions for a healthy child is a half teaspoon mixed with 2 oz. water or juice then double every fifteen minutes until a watery stool. Start at 2 teaspoons for a child who is not healthy. When it becomes watery, taper back to a healthy stool.

Magnesium can be used as a constipation remedy, gradually increasing the dose to restore proper bowel movements.[238]

Molasses and milk enema.[239] I learned about this gentle treatment from Toni Kaplan, a nurse supporting my kids' recovery, as a way to add water to the stool. An enema with 12 oz. each milk or substitute milk, and molasses can help when your child is squatting and uncomfortable.

Common Sense, Practical Ways to Detoxify

Don't just remove toxicity from the body but figure out the source. Remove dental amalgams, test your water for lead, don't eat fish and avoid mercury.

Epsom Salt bath is slow, calming way to detoxify the body through the skin. Make sure the Epsom salt is good quality without extra additives. Use a cup of Epsom salt, a tablespoon of baking soda and a drop of lavender essential oil, and take a bath for 20 minutes for an adult. Magnesium will help calm the child, get a good night sleep and can help with constipation.

Zeolite will trap and remove heavy metals from the body and will also help the body to remove radiation. It can be in a powdered or liquid form. As a powdered form, it's gritty and I recommend mixing with a strong juice like grape juice and drinking quickly with a straw. It settles at the bottom of the glass and will need frequent stirring.

Ion Cleanse: These are chemically reactive and produced many beneficial ions that you breathe near a beach or a waterfall. This is a more expensive form of detoxifying the body. You can purchase one at amajordifference.com.

Common Tests

There are many blood, stool, and urine tests that people can take to identify the medical problems associated with autism and its symptoms. I am only going to mention three popular ones because to list them all would be too much. Secondly, not everyone needs every single test, though most doctors that specialize in this treatment will do numerous tests in the beginning to figure out your child individually.

Porphyrin Testing. Porphyrins are proteins that calculate the heme in the urine which transports oxygen, energy and detoxification. The toxicity may not be present in the blood, hair or urine and has be drawn out of the organs of the body first. The test is a six-hour urine collection to compare the sample before and after chelation to get these to the urine where it would be if the body could detoxify correctly. Genova Diagnostics does this test.

Comprehensive Stool Analysis This will measure bacteria, parasites, inflammation, viruses, food sensitivities and pathogens in the gut. This is a stool sample taken into a small vial for analysis on two separate days, twelve hours apart. Great Plains Laboratories does this test.

IGG Food Allergy Candida Test. This is an immunoglobulin test also by Great Plains to see if 93 different food allergies are a contributing factor for people with disorders like autism,

ADHD, cystic fibrosis, rheumatoid arthritis and epilepsy among others. It will also test for candida which is associated with autism, MS and chronic fatigue. This test can be done at home and shipped to a lab.

Behaviors

Toxicity, gut problems, vaccines and viruses can contribute to problematic behaviors. Sometimes these are best solved with therapy to teach the child how to cope and what to do in each situation.

They not only need to learn how to cope with sensitivities or loud noises or strong smells, but appropriate ways to handle them. A team effort is needed from doctors, medical professionals and therapists to understand what the child is sensitive to, as well as what to do when he is around that chemical or toxicity causing the problem.

Not every child has these behaviors but they are common for many on the spectrum.

Some behaviors are diagnosed as EMOTIONAL or MENTAL, but they nonetheless might have their roots in an unhealthy gut.

TICS and OCD

TICS or spasmodic twitching in the facial area, and some obsessive-compulsive disorders can sometimes be linked to autoimmune gut disorders.[240] For example, Strep, a contagious bacterial disease, enters from the throat, but can result in an autoimmune disease called PANDAS (Pediatric Autoimmune Neuropsychiatric Disorder Associated with Streptococcus), with added TICS and OCD symptoms. The child also may have inflamed tonsils or inflammation.

General Neuropsychiatric Symptoms

Anger/Depression/frustration

This can be psychological but at root, it is also a frustration of not being able to express or communicate correctly. Though a therapist or school counselor can help with coping strategies or therapy to handle this emotional overload as it occurs, there are also environmental and medical problems that coexist.

Allergies, bacteria, parasites and GMOS can all create what we now call mental symptoms and a disorder called PANDAS can cause moodiness, anxiety, and irritability.[241] Allergies can cause moodiness, suicidal thoughts and depression.[242]

Don't touch what hurts

Skin sensitivities make the skin physically painful. This child does not like to be touched or the clothes burn or itch, or one child told me that "rain felt like fire." The child may remove clothes that are itchy because they contain chemicals like formaldehyde that make them so. Or the child is allergic to the fabric. For people who are sensitive to chemicals, the smell, the feel, the fabric itself will hurt and they will remove what hurts, even if you touching them is what hurts. Lisa Marks Smith, injured by the flu shot explains it as feeling like a burn patient. Physical touch is painful.

Fight or Flight

This behavior becomes another way for children to avoid what bothers them. People on the spectrum react the way anyone would to avoid something uncomfortable or overbearing like a loud noise. They can shut it out by putting their hands on their ears, they can turn off the noise, or fight the person who makes it, or they can leave the room. It's a non-verbal way to remove yourself from a bad situation, like trying to teach algebra in the middle of a war. Remove the war, then they can learn.

Stimming or self-stimulation,

This is the child's way of coping with the battleground. What do you do before an important speech to the CEO? You pace, you drum your pencil, you squirm, or fidget. Kids on the spectrum do this all the time because the world itself is that stressful. Sometimes, even when good things happen, kids will fidget even more.

Screaming

Think of screaming as a signal for being overwhelmed or in pain, as an inappropriate way of not handling the battleground well. Pay attention to what your child is doing, what part of his body he's holding, or focusing on. If screaming is an expression of gut pain, the source could be inflammation, viruses, toxicity, bowel problems or infections. For example, people with chronic constipation describe it as if an anvil landed on their stomach. Screaming communicates this pain.

Brain fog

This just simply becoming forgetful, short-term memory loss, forgetting tests, walking into a room and forgetting why.

Appears Drugged

He appears glassy eyed, and falling over like a drunk. He may also steal food, cram the food into the mouth, and behave as if he has insatiable hunger or thirst. The gastrointestinal system malfunctioning and food is not digested and it creates an opiate like effect as if they were intoxicated. Peptides passing through the leaky gut or intestinal permeability causing the child to behave as if drugged, because the food passes through the intestinal membrane to the central nervous system. Gluten and casein can have this effect, hence the reason for many kids to begin the gluten and casein free diet. This is the opiate theory of autism.[243] The gut damage can be the result of toxicity, vaccines, viruses or all three.

Head banging

Like screaming, head banging is an expression of pain. I've spoken to recovering kids who describe headaches that hurt so much that they feel like banging their head on the floor. Migraines, headaches from allergies, or encephalitis (inflammation in the brain), can be associated with what you eat.

Ibuprofen can block pain temporarily, and it does help but not if you keep eating what is causing the headache, or injecting it via vaccines.

One common problem is that Monosodium Glutamate (MSG), a food additive in most processed products, can activate TRESK, a gene that causes migraines. Advil, a common pain reliever, can block glutamates, solving the problem temporarily. However, avoiding MSG improves gut health and prevents these headaches in some children, improving behavior because pain is reduced.

Scratching

Scratching is sometimes simply a reaction to an itch, and itching is an example of allergies or gut imbalance. The child not only may need something to relieve the symptom of the itch, but to also pay attention to the allergies or parasite that might make one scratch. Parasites like hookworm or ancylostomiasis, which live in the intestines, or food allergies are also common. You might see eggs or other parasite evidence in your child's poop. You can also track scratching symptoms by keeping a food diary and linking the behavior to the kind of food they've recently eaten, gradually treating the itch by correcting the child's diet. Common allergies like gluten sensitivity can cause dermatitis herpetiformis, an itchy bumpy rash from eating gluten.[244] (For more on allergies, see Sarah's story, *The Sensitive Child.*)

Tools to Track Success
Autism Treatment Evaluation Checklist (http://www.surveygizmo.com/s3/1329619/Autism-Treatment-Evaluation-Checklist-revised)

This list will give you a snapshot when you first begin and again after evaluating treatment to see what worked and what did not. You can compare behaviors now to what they were when you started treatment. The more symptoms the child has the higher the score in this checklist. You want a lower score to show signs of recovery.

Use Appendix L's simple behavior chart to help your process.

Add to it the diet, possible contributing factor and time and place of behavior. See if you can see a pattern of where and when it occurred, paying attention to chemical and physical patterns in the environment. This is not to diagnose, but simply to take notes.

In the beginning of your healing journey, it helps to keep a food diary to understand which foods may be linked to a behavior which may show a pattern. Sometimes the behaviors still occur but not as often. It's important to note how long they happen, and if the child can self-regulate and calm himself or learn to cope effectively. There is room for notes as to notice patterns. Was it a food, time of day, location? When and where does behavior occur?

Helpful Sites for More Information

MAPS (http://www.medmaps.org/clinician-directory/)

This stands for Medical Academy of Pediatric Special Needs. Here is a list of doctors who have been trained in the underlying issues of autism so that you can begin medical treatment individualized to fit your family needs.

Autism 360 (http://autism360.org/)

This site tracks your child's needs to a region to match up with another local parent with similar needs. This way you can swap resources, doctors and offer each other advice.

Generation Rescue (http://www.generationrescue.org/newly-diagnosed/)

This is another site that links you with a local parent to find resources. If you are a knowledgeable parent, you can be a "rescue angel" and help someone nearby.

What You Can Do In The School Setting: Advice For Team Building And Successful IEPs

Assembling Your Team

For a parent to know how to handle his child needs, the parent needs a team of specialists who can work together, and understand the medical issues and behavioral issues are one and the same. An effective team will understand how medical needs can affect behaviors and vice versa. Behaviorists also teach the child coping skills, and support their learning process so they can react more appropriately and help others understand what they are trying to communicate.

A team needs to include medical and behavioral professionals. The behavioral portion may be people such as social workers, psychologists, psychiatrists, therapists such as vision, ABA, physical, and occupational. The medical portion may be allergists, pediatricians, naturopaths, dentists, a pediatrician, family doctor or a naturopath who understands your child's medical needs. You may also see Lyme Specialists, mold removal technicians, dieticians, gastroenterologists, and neurologists.

The schools look at your child from an academic, task-based perspective. There are behavior therapists on staff to figure out if there is something that the school can do to lessen the child's stress so that he can learn properly. Sometimes the problem is behavioral but sometimes it's medical. A parent with a special needs kid will spend more time and effort than any full-time job taking their child to the entire medical team and must connect them to each other so they understand each person's part in the child's care. Keep notes on what happens and when and some people have their own personal medical file to take from one specialist to another. Ask each one to keep their recommendations written down because sometimes you need to take the written information and bring it to someone else on your team and they all listen to you the parent more often if you have a note from a professional backing up everything you tell them.

Both parents need to be on the home team. One parent as a researcher and the other to take notes or budget for certain remedies. Both parents decide ahead of time when meeting with the specialist as having a "job" at the meeting. Sometimes having a male voice in the room can be beneficial when most of the time the specialists are female.

The medical team may know very well that the behavioral needs are caused by medical issues but the parent then should get notes from the medical team to give to the school because the school hires or fires teachers or even gets penalized or fined because they child can't or won't complete a task. The parent is juggling to stop the behaviors so the child can complete a task with the medical problems getting in the way.

Your child's medical needs that get in the way of his education should be taught to every teacher, social worker, or therapist that works in the school setting. Bring your information with you to the school for personnel to read and offer them information. Some schools have a parent library. You can offer them information for not just parents but teachers too. The education for teachers does not include any medical issues and at best an overview of what the behaviors are, but not how medical issues can affect academics.

Recommended Information for Your IEP

This information should be added in your IEP:

- Diets and their consequences. Does the child vomit or have diarrhea after eating off the diet? When you tell the school this, they are less likely to let the child cheat knowing he's on school grounds.
- Modified changes in chemicals, air cleaners, school supplies, foods, so that the child is not trying to learn in an environment that is overwhelming or can even make him sick.

- This includes things like awareness of toxic or allergy stimulants:
  - Astroturf
  - Cleaning Products
  - Mold
  - Dust
  - Chemicals
  - Peanuts
- If the child can communicate well enough to advocate for himself what he can eat, teach him what is in a vaccine to communicate that as well.
- The school team needs to be aware of toxicity that effects learning and thinking. Lead, fluoride, mold, allergies, and vaccine status will lower the child's ability to learn and think and answer questions correctly.

Rules for Navigating Your IEP

Here are my rules for getting through the Individual Education Plan and living to tell the tale.

1. Always bring someone with you. You are part of the team but sometimes it feels like they are lecturing or pushing you to do certain things and it feels like you against them. It is nice to have someone on your side. Sometimes, if that person is male, they will unfortunately listen more attentively.

2. As a two-person team bring a list of what you need from the school in writing 24 hours in advance. If you have things you need to include in the IEP you must submit it in writing twenty-four hours in advance. It's like a counter-proposal. Bring your information to compare with what the school has already decided your child needs.

3. As a practice, notify the school that you will be recording the IEP meeting because you are terrible at taking notes. If you record the meeting, so will they and become accountable for what they say and do. Don't make a big deal about this because it's intimidating to the school.

4. Always bring a document by a professional about why your child does what he does. If your child has chronic fatigue due to Lyme or turns his papers in late due to poor executive functioning send in a letter written by that therapist, medical doctor or whatever you need to explain the behavior. You cannot simply explain what happened at your last doctor's appointment. It should be a letter signed by the doctor (even if you wrote it), but on his letterhead with his signature. This documentation should explain what the behavior is, and then what the doctor or therapist's opinion is about what is causing it. This will force the people in the IEP to put in a plan in place to correct the behavior instead of just dismissing, ignoring or even punishing or rewarding him for it.

5. If your child has some behavior issues where he has been suspended or expelled, get a therapist who knows your child well to call the school or write a letter to explain these behaviors. A good therapist can get your child out of trouble especially if this issue is due to a disability and you can document it. Even if your child has a therapist he sees only periodically, and this therapist knows him well, he can offer expert support. A school that suspends your child with disruptive behavior will tell you to find a therapist anyway, and if you don't have one that knows your child well, you may have to settle very quickly for one who may not be your first choice.

6. Get a Behavior Intervention Plan or BIP. If you do this at the first sign of a behavior issue, this can save you a lot of hassle. A behavior specialist assigned to the school will do an analysis to find out why your child does what he does so that the teachers are not in fact rewarding your child instead of punishing him. If your child doesn't want to do certain things and has a meltdown, the teachers might send him to the Principal's office where he sits and doesn't have to do what he didn't want to do in the first place. Also, the behaviorist will find ways to motivate your child.

7. Your child has the right for a Free and Appropriate Public Education. This is known as FAPE. He cannot be expelled from school because of a disability. The school should have a place for him to go to get an education. Therefore, autism schools are popping up everywhere as a place to put our kids on the spectrum. If your child is put into a facility like this, he still has the right to learn basic skills like math and reading and you can make sure that this happens. These other schools are not meant to be a babysitting service. If there are life skills to learn or job skills to learn in a facility like that and your child can learn them than you can get this to happen.

8. Make sure the goals are clear, measurable and accountable. Your IEP goals are not simply a list of behaviors. These are concrete action plans as to how to fix it and who is responsible to make sure that happens. Make sure that there is a way for the goal to be met and someone who will take responsibility for meeting it.

If the goal says "teacher assigned rubric" that means your teacher can do whatever they want to meet the goal. How do you know whether their method is working if it isn't written down? Some teachers are naturally skilled at adapting strategies to help your child but others aren't. If your child has many teachers, they all use a different "teacher assigned rubric" and therefore there may be 4 different teachers with completely different ways of accommodating your child. Unfortunately, sometimes when the child doesn't meet the goal, the parent or the child himself is blamed, although the problem comes because there is no consistency in the child's education plan. If the goal is ongoing, leave it on the IEP, to let teachers know it's a problem. Be clear and consistent.

Types of things the behavior specialist can do for you.

ABC: Antecedent-Behavior-Consequence (a method of tracking targeted behaviors) (ABC Data is used to help us to identify the function of the behavior. We usually observe the behavior (B) and implement a consequence (C) however; we often miss identifying the antecedent (A). That antecedent drives the function of that observed behavior so we can "label it" as escape, access, attention and avoidance AND most importantly, develop a replacement behavior.

Applied Behavior Analysis which is a method to reward your child to learn certain activities with positive behavior modification.

If all else fails, hire an advocate. This is an attorney who will come to the IEP and fight for you. This is very expensive and a last resort but if your advocate can get you a detailed plan from the start, this plan can be adjusted over the years to make sure your child gets what he needs in the school. This is necessary for a child who has discipline problems especially if those problems are due to his disability.

Types of Things an Advocate can do for you.

If your child is not receiving services or the school wants your child to have certain services but asks that you pay for them at home, you can hire an advocate to request that these services are provided in the school setting.

She will take the history of your child, meet and observe and talk to him and make recommendations for services, rewrite your IEP with a counter proposal of services and offer you feedback.

This is expensive but worth it if your child is not getting a Free and Appropriate Public Education. (FAPE)

If you want to get through your child's school career, you need to speak the lingo. If you can speak the school jargon to school administrators, staff, case managers and social workers you will open doors and get the services you need faster but you need to be able to ask for them in the way they need to hear it.

You also need to know ahead of time what services the school has available. If you can speak the lingo, you will be able to ask for these services. Some schools have a lot of services but they won't offer them unless you ask. Sometimes schools wait until the behavior has escalated beyond their control instead of being proactive and stopping the behavior before it begins.

Labels You Might Encounter at Your IEP Meeting

ADD: Attention Deficit Disorder

A child with this label might have help for organization or executive functioning. If your child needs speech as well, then get a second label for speech.

ADHD, or MBD: Attention Deficit Hyperactivity Disorder or Minimum Brain Dysfunction which is the older label for ADHD.

A child with this label is fidgety and squirmy. He needs movement and perhaps this movement helps him to think better. He might get help with the organization but the school wants control and for him to sit still. The school is not allowed to suggest medication but they might.

APD: Auditory Processing Disorder

Does the child understand what was being said to him? Can he overcome background noises that may be distracting or overbearing?

AS: Asperger's Syndrome, also called HFA (Higher Functioning Autism)

ASD: Autism Spectrum Disorder

Your child must have this diagnosis from a doctor. He must have impairments in speech and communication and social skills.

BP: Bipolar or sometimes called MD (Manic Depressive)

This is a child who is hyper one day and depressed the next. Read The Hyper Child or The Depressed or Angry Child. Your child's behavior may have many underlying causes and many medical issues. This must be diagnosed by a medical professional. In the school setting, the modifications the school needs would be to figure out what makes him hyper or depressed and is he further exposed during school. Is the school rewarding the behavior? The clues are to figure out medical, as well as his sensory and emotional issues that might create certain behaviors and what motivates the child to discontinue behavior.

DD: Developmental Disabilities

EI: Early Intervention

ECSE: Early Childhood Special Education

These are all labels for very young children perhaps too young to be labeled as autism or Asperger's. If your child gets diagnosed very young, see if he can get an autism diagnosis because it might qualify him for more services at school.

ED: Emotionally Disturbed

HoH: Hard of Hearing

Does the child need headphones, a hearing aid or any other modification?

ID: Intellectual Disability or MD for Mental Retardation

This might be a child who scored poorly on an IQ test. Make sure he has proper accommodations to take the test. Some children can score higher if they type their answers for example. Children can sometimes score low on this test but they may know more than the test reveals because they had no accommodations.

LD: Learning Disability. (These are things like Dyslexia or Dyscalculia.)

These are ways that your child sees numbers or letters in a jumbled order.

LFA: Low-Functioning Autism

This is defined as autism occurring with mental retardation, e.g. w/ IQ lower than 70.

LLD: Language-based Learning Disability

MDO: Major Depressive Disorder

This is a child clinically diagnosed as depressed.

MH: Multiple Handicapped

This is a child with more than one diagnosis.

MH: Mental Health

MPD: Multiple Personality Disorder

MR: Mental Retardation, IQ < 70 (Now ID)

NOS: Not Otherwise Specified, sometimes called PDD (Persuasive Developmental Disorder) and PDD-NOS (Persuasive Developmentally Disorder Not Otherwise Specified)

This is a fancy way of saying that your child meets some of the criteria for autism but not all. He may still need some accommodations in the school setting.

NLD or NVLD: Non-Verbal Learning Disability

OCD and TD: Obsessive-Compulsive Disorder

TS: Tourette's syndrome

This is a child who has trouble changing routine. This is a child full of yeast, or possibly suffering from PANDAS or Lyme. Many kids with OCD also have tics or Tourette's.

ODD, PTSD, or SED: This stand for Oppositional-Defiant Disorder, Post-Traumatic Stress Disorder, and Severely Emotionally Disturbed.

Read the Depressed or Angry Child. This is a child who needs a Behavior Intervention Plan to be modified or changed to figure out why this happens and create a plan to help your child deal with his stress in a school setting. This may be sensory problem or a feeling of being overwhelmed. Breaking big tasks into small ones or scheduling time may help. Removing the child from whatever is causing the sensory issues may help calm him. If something is too loud or too smelly for example, he can't concentrate and if he can't tell you this, he melts down. Nonverbal kids with sensory issues can be tough to figure out because they can't tell you what is bothering them. A computer aided device where the child can communicate pain or smells or sensory issues in school will let the child tell teachers directly so they make corrections in the school setting.

OHI or POHI: Other Health Impaired, or Physical or Otherwise Health Impaired.

SID: Sensory Integration Dysfunction, also referred to as SI, or DSI

This child is very sensory oriented and his meltdowns may indicate he can't process things that are too loud or smell for example.

SIB: Self-Injurious Behavior

The child bangs his head, for example. In a school setting, monitor what he was doing before this occurs and see if there is anything sensory or emotionally overloading for him.

Tests Your School Might Offer to Determine the Best Services for Your Child

DAS: Differential Abilities Scales (an early childhood educational evaluation)

EPSDT: Early Periodic Screening Diagnosis and Treatment

IEE: Independent Educational Evaluation

GAF: Global Assessment of Functioning scale (used in psychiatric evaluations to state level of functioning)

PIQ: Performance Intelligence Quotient

WAIS: Wechsler Adult Intelligence Scale (an IQ test)

WISC: Wechsler Intelligence Scale for Children (an IQ test)

W-J-R: Woodcock-Johnson Revised (a psycho-educational test)

VIQ: Verbal IQ

Pay attention to how the tests are done. Does the child have trouble writing but the measure for success in a test is writing with a pencil? See if perhaps he might do better with a computer. Some children need the tests read verbally. Some children need glasses or a hearing aid or some other accommodation to be able to do well on the test. Many children don't get these accommodations and do not do as well on these tests as they could.

Therapies and Interventions Schools Might Propose

APE: Adaptive Physical Education

Read the Exhausted Child. If your child has Lyme or Chronic Fatigue, a thyroid or a mitochondrial dysfunction, get him a note from the doctor to discontinue activities he is too tired to do. The APE teacher can make changes to the curriculum to make your child personal goals instead of following the rest of the class.

BIP: Behavior Intervention Plan

This is a plan by a behavior specialist to determine why a behavior occurs and what to do about it. Don't wait until the child has multiple discipline problems to do this if you know there is a disability or medical reason. Do this at the first sign of a behavior problem. This makes the school accountable for correcting and modifying the behaviors at school, and not blaming parents.

ESY: Extended School Year

If your child has a poor short-term memory, sometimes he needs to continue school during the summer. If he is likely to forget issues quickly this might be an option.

ESL: English as a Second Language

Parents speak a language other than English at home. The child not only has to overcome his disability but learn a new language too.

IEP or 504: Individualized Education Plan

This is a plan for accommodations in the school setting. A child gets a 504 instead of an IEP when he has a learning disability, an allergy or perhaps needs minor accommodations but doesn't fit into autism or any related category.

LRE: Least Restrictive Environment

Put the child in a place where he is the most accepted in the school setting. If he can be placed in a general education setting and still get his accommodations met, then this is the LRE.

OT: Occupational Therapy;
PT: Physical Therapy;
SP Speech Therapy

A therapist is needed to help a child who can help meet his goals if he needs help writing or in PE or cannot do certain activities.

PLEP and PLOP: Present Levels of Educational Performance or Present Level of Performance.

What does your child already know how to do? Schools tend to focus on what your child cannot do, but sometimes using skills your child already knows, teachers can help your child with things that he lacks.

Sped: Special Education

PTI: Parent Training and Information Center

This is a school library for educational needs.

Legal Terms

These are your child's rights and yours. Before you sign anything make sure that you read them. Many schools make you sign a document saying that you received these documents. Read them.

ESEA: Elementary & Secondary Education Act

FERPA: Federal Educational Rights and Privacy Act

IDEA: Individuals with Disabilities Education Act

LEA: Local Education Agency (the school district)

Government Agencies

NAMI: National Association for the Mentally Ill

NICHCY: National Information Centers for Children and Youth with Disabilities

NIH: National Institute for Health

OCR: Office of Civil Rights **OSEP:** Office of Special Education Programs (located Washington, DC)

OSERS: Office of Special Education and Rehabilitative Services

P&A: Protection & Advocacy

SD: School District

SEA: State Education Agency

People Who May Work with your Child

Case Manager

This is your main contact when things go wrong and the person who can fix it. Get to know this person and email or call as issues arise.

Social Worker

MDT: Multi-Disciplinary Team; TSS Therapeutic Support Staff.

OT-Occupational Therapist

SIPT: Sensory Integration and Praxis Text

SLP: Speech-Language Pathologist

TSS: Therapeutic Support Staff

Other Medical References

PDR: Physician's Desk Reference

PET: Positron Emission Tomography

This is a brain scan that can be used for diagnosis of neurologically-based disorders.

Rx: Prescription

SSRI: Selective Serotonin Reuptake Inhibitors

This is a class of medications, including Prozac, Zoloft, Paxil, and Luvox. These drugs correct a chemical imbalance in the brain. As you read the part about the gut, you see that that dopamine and serotonin are in the gut as well as the brain and so the gut plays a role in these chemical imbalances. There may be a long list of things once thought to be purely a brain disorder that show dysfunction somewhere else in the body and should be medically treated accordingly.

TEACCH: Treatment and Education of Autistic and Related Communication Disorders

Frequent Mistakes Schools Make About Our Kids

1. Create goals that are not measurable and then make you, the parent, accountable for any success of failure.

These goals need to be broken into small tasks and accountable to someone at school. There needs to be a clear action plan on how to fix it and what you are doing about it.

2. Reward the child for misbehavior.

If your child melts down for sensory issues and this can include emotions of people in the room, removing that child from the situation can be calming but it's also a reward. If your child knows that he will be removed from a situation that is too loud or emotional and he doesn't want to be there, then some schools have a time out area but this child needs this to calm down. The child needs someone to talk to him to figure out what the sensory issue was and to fix it and not just put him in isolation and to learn how and what caused the behavior.

3. No behavior plan in place.

The child just gets written up or sent to the Principal's office without anyone figuring out what happened.

4. Child was not given clear instructions.

"Put your stuff away" is not a clear instruction. The teacher sometimes gives vague directions like this, an overwhelmed child who does not know how to organize might take that to mean shove his stuff in the desk. A better instruction is to say, "Put your books in this pile. Put your scissors in this supply bin. Put your crayons in the box." Your child thinks he is following your teacher's directions because they were muddled. If this needs to be spelled out in the IEP that the child needs clear directions, then please do this and don't assume your teacher has had any training in autism. A general education teacher has had minimal training because this is not part of the general educational curriculum for teachers. It should be.

5. Teachers are unaware of physical or medical limitations.

If your child has a physical issue that limits his learning process. Bring a note from a doctor that specifies how and why it limits education. If you just tell the teacher, he will not have clear instructions as to what accommodations he needs. If you have a note from the doctor, it is every teacher's responsibility to read it and not to punish the child because he can't do something. The medical note is there for a reason. Read it.

6. Teachers only giving worst-case scenarios.

Some teachers will threaten or yell to get the children to comply. This will backfire for a special needs child because they tend to be quite literal and panic. The child may feel the yelling is directed at him when it might be for the whole class. The child takes the emotions personally, even if he did nothing wrong and then think that this teacher hates him. He needs to know that this is not the case. Positive reinforcement works better.

*7. Teachers use the word **don't** too much.*

"Don't do this" and "don't do that" are confusing for our kids. Tell the child what you do want him to do. If the child is standing on a chair, instead of saying, "You could fall and break your neck." The child is literally thinking he will fall and break his neck. It is better to say, "Sit with your hands folded." Reward the students behaving correctly. Kids on the spectrum take things very literally and saying things like this will terrify them.

8. Teachers who use too many metaphors.

People on the spectrum sometimes do not understand metaphors. If you tell them it's raining cats and dogs, the child will literally look up in the sky for cats and dogs. Be clear and give direct instructions. Inferring correct behavior is hard for our kids. Help and explain metaphors or give them a metaphor dictionary to learn a new phrase every day.

9. Present too many ways to solve a math problem or other challenge.

If one way is working for them and the answer is correct, let them be. It's good to teach them multiple ways to solve problems but let them use the method they prefer. Sometimes kids are obsessed with solving things a certain way but that's because it's how they learn and it's okay.

10. Require kids to conform to standards that don't account for their synesthesia.

Synesthesia means they see numbers with colors and shapes, or have another sense activated with language, music or other stimulation. If they want to solve their math problem with colored pencils, let them. It won't be the way they were taught to solve the problem but if the answer is correct, let them do it this way. This would be hard to put in a curriculum because for example every child may see the number four a different color or shape which is hard to teach in a classroom. This child may be brilliant at math but he should do it the way he knows and then re do it the way he was taught and it can be confusing. Teachers should at the very least be taught what synesthesia is.

11. Refuse proper accommodations when administering tests.

Children may be much smarter than what the IQ tests allow. Give them space and the proper techniques to figure it out.

12. Disregard necessary conditions to support openness and focus for kids with sensory issues.

If the test has loud sounds or bright lights, the child is in defense mode and may be trying to overcome these issues. He may not be able to concentrate and may not do as well.

Part 6: Decoding Other Behaviors Using this Guide: More Stories

Introduction

I had some difficulty with this book because it is simply wrong to say one solution works for every child, or that if you do this one thing it will "cure" autism. The stories in this book focused on a process that has worked for many of us, thinking about just one behavior and what was done to correct it. I explained useful ideas that helped my children or the people I interviewed, not to present a cure for autism but to show the importance of common medical issues, noting what behaviors disappeared. I also used the difference in how I felt before and after my own medical treatments to write these stories, because physical problems like allergies and toxicity run in families. I think that autistic kids may be thinking the same things that I was but they are unable to articulate the problem, or name the solution. While I could complain, and do something about it, they could not. I want parents, teachers and therapists to understand what that kind of stress feels like, so that it can be avoided and kids can work at their own energy level and not to suggest that every kid has the same amount of energy and may need frequent breaks to recover.

Instead of writing a dry list of symptoms and lists like most books about the same subjects written by doctors, I wrote this in a story format, so you can read it quickly in an afternoon and understand your child, and we can work as a team to understand our kids' thoughts and feelings a little bit better, speaking about each symptom in situations of people I know or interviewed.

Next, I'll tell more stories to help you decode different kinds of behaviors, so you can have even more information and support.

The Sensitive Child
MICHAEL: The Empathic Child.

Michael wore his half zip pullover mostly unzipped because the zipper was cold and scratchy. He could not put them on already zipped because then they would not fit over his rather large head. His pullovers either had zippers or he would wear button down shirts to fit over his head. The sleeves were too long and covered his hands. When Michael was bored or he needed to calm himself, he chewed on his sleeves. He didn't just chew on his sleeves he gnawed as if his sleeve was a piece of gum. His sleeves usually had a hole about a half an inch below where the sleeve began and Michael had a habit of putting his thumb in the hole which made the hole even bigger.

If Michael wore anything that wasn't soft cotton, he was very itchy. Johnson's Baby Shampoo burned his skin and his ivory soap gave him hives. He was always barefoot because shoes felt uncomfortable and unnecessary and Michael would take them off at the first opportunity. Michael just preferred to go barefoot. His teeth were yellow because he wouldn't allow his mother to brush them because the toothbrush felt like a soldering iron on his teeth.

He liked quiet areas and kept to himself but not because he was anti-social or that he didn't like certain people but because people often had one expression but felt something totally different. People would have a smile on their face and not feel happy. He thought they were being fake. They often asked him, "How are you?" but didn't really care because it was a greeting not really wanting to know how he was. They wore perfume that smelled like petroleum which to him was stinky and nauseating.

Michael had a sense about other people and he knew their moods, their emotions and who they really were without ever having a conversation with them. He thought they had empathy with him the same way so therefore he didn't need to talk. The others around him were only thinking about themselves and not about Michael at all but that's not what he thought. He had deep empathy and profound thoughts to feel others emotions very deeply but he didn't always want to know why and felt like he had to ask. Something innocent about Michael drew people to him even complete strangers told him things they never told anyone else because he knew their emotions deeply, and he cried when they cried. He couldn't separate their emotions from his own and truly felt them in his heart.

The problem was that being that empathic also drained his energy being around other people. For him to recharge, refocus and concentrate on the task at hand he needed to be alone without other people's emotions interfering in his life. People might call him snobbish, shy, or overemotional but his gift was his empathy. This could get in the way of tests and make him as nervous as the whole room or as excited, depending on how people were feeling. He didn't have to guess; he knew. But he needed to spend time alone to recharge and get away from the negativity and people needed to understand that.

He liked to spend time with babies because they were the most honest about their emotions. Sometimes walking into a room with an adult or other child feeling angry or sad was too much for him, and he would have to leave the room to regain control of his own emotions. His connection to others was deep but instead of being closer to them he felt further apart. He knew exactly what their emotions felt like because he could feel them too. Michael would tell his mother great emotional intellectual things like a little Plato. Michael was a wise man but he was only six. He asked her thoughtful questions like "What happens when you die? Do dogs go to heaven? Do plants have feelings too?" When he asked the questions, he already knew the answers. He had his response prepared, and he just wanted to see what his mother would say. Here is what he said once: "Each body has a soul, including dogs, and even plants. That's why we pray before we eat, asking the animal or plant's permission to consume it."

His mother would hear him say these great words of wisdom and smile as if she were watching him preach a great sermon but his great intellectual and emotional intelligence did not translate to elementary school because in some areas he was lacking. Those things dragged him down and made him fail. Michael could see colors and shapes in his head that were complicated math calculations, because he had synesthesia which meant he could use colors and shapes to define numbers. He couldn't "show his work" and did not understand the math without vibrant colors. Five was brilliant blue circle and seven was a pale green rectangle. He couldn't explain how he had his answers but he was usually right. His tests didn't reflect his ability and showing his work the way teachers told him slowed him down and he was put in remedial math because there was no math teacher that taught the way that he thought about numbers. Math was art.

Michael had a lot of trouble eating because eating hot food was out of the question. He would not touch food just out of the oven or the slightest bit too warm. He had to eat everything ice cold because the hot or warm food felt like a second-degree burn. His mom had to cook the food and put it in the freezer before dinner so it was cold enough to eat. He craved ice cream, ice, and preferred cold pizza. Michael had cavities all right next to each other on the right side so Michael's head felt like someone was pushing him to the right when he ate anything but especially if he was eating something hot.

In school, kids knew Michael would cry for just about anything but a loud noise would completely set him off. He would hold his ears and scream at the fire alarm to the point where the teachers were taking him outside ten minutes before the drill to lessen the noise and he could wear noise-canceling headphones. In fact, if he could, Michael would wear those headphones all the time because when the whole class was talking, it was not just deafening, but Michael felt all the kids' happiness, sadness and anger all at the same time which felt overpowering and almost nauseating. He needed to clear out the emotions of others as well as their jabbering. He needed solitude.

Michael had a superior IQ but he couldn't hear his own thoughts because the other children's thoughts and feelings were too much. When they were talking, he couldn't tell if anyone was talking to him because it sounded like a World Wrestling Shouting Match with the whole world yelling at once. In the right quiet one on one environment, Michael could thrive but a room of thirty screaming kids wasn't it. He did not qualify as mentally retarded because his IQ was tested at 130. But he needed quiet to work, and the smells that other people had from their soaps, lotions and antibacterial hand wash to their shampoo made him physically gag, toothpaste made him wince and sometimes the art supplies like clay made his hands itch. The uncomfortable feelings that were around him all the time were unbearable and it was very difficult to cancel them out and focus on his schoolwork which he thought was boring, so he didn't score well on tests.

Michael's mom spent a lot of time learning from friends on Facebook where to find a more natural shampoo, hand lotion, toothpaste, or soap that didn't give him hives or make him itch. She had to send his own soaps to school and more natural school supplies. She had to search hard because his current soap made his hands raw from the soap he used and his hair itched from his shampoo. Michael was diagnosed with Bipolar Disorder because sometimes he was hyper and sometimes he was depressed and it all depended on the toxins in his environment for that day. He also was diagnosed with a developmental delay because he had allergic reactions to different chemicals he was touching, smelling or eating. His eyes glazed over with dark circles under them. His cheeks were red like they had just been slapped. His lips were puffy and so were his eyes. He was not anaphylactic to peanuts but he was having a reaction. He also had rashes that came and went with each vaccination. His doctor said he had a "measles like" reaction to the MMR vaccine but that it couldn't be measles since he just had the shot. Most of Michael's behaviors were directly related to his environment which needed to be cleaned up for him to thrive in school.

Tools for Michael's Family

Michael has a chemical sensitivity. His need for solitude can be self-medicating for him to remove himself from chemicals that are physically making him sick. Read and Google all ingredients of food as well as soap, shampoo, hand sanitizer. Even the dough used in school can be toxic for a kid like Michael. Here is a good place to search for natural products. http://www.ewg.org/

Some experts say that people on the spectrum stay away from large crowds because they have no empathy but in Michael's case he has empathy in abundance. "The Intense World Theory" by the Brain-Mind Institute proposes that the progression of the disorder is proposed to be driven by overly strong reactions to experiences that drive the brain to a hyper-preference and overly selective state, which becomes more extreme with each new experience and may be particularly accelerated by emotionally charged experiences and trauma. "That means the child is more empathic, not less, and feels every smell, touch, taste, sound, and emotion more intensely not less and that they can become over stimulated and overpowered by these experiences. Michael is an example of what a child who sees the world so intensely might do or say."

Michael's world is still full of people who use toxic products and sometimes if their perfume or soap gives him a headache he may need to stay away. This is not anti-social behavior; it's a chemical sensitivity. For Michael to be able to function, he can either learn how to tell others about the cologne they are using or he can sometimes go to a naturopath to treat these reactions to chemicals like an allergy and sometimes these reactions can change an entire personality. Read the book "Is This Your Child?" by Doris Rapp.

Michael had Synesthesia, a condition where you associate multiple stimulus like letters and numbers with other senses, like colors, shapes, smells and tastes. Kids like Michael can use shapes and colors to do math or learn music. It's different for everyone, so this cannot be taught, but some kids can be amazing mathematicians or musicians because of this sensibility.

Kids with a high mercury level can feel sensory input like sound unbearable. Lisa Marks Smith explains that after her flu shot, sounds were "equally loud." That's what Michael was experiencing. You can do sensory integration therapy to cope. Michael also had a mouth full of dental amalgams causing a mouth sensitivity.

Read the book Dental Mercury Detox: A Health Information Book to Answer Questions You May Have on Countering the Effects of Dental Mercury Exposure, by Sam Ziff. Also, go to the International Academy of Oral Medicine and Toxicology, where you will find information about mercury and toxins in dentistry, and a list of mercury free dentists.

Keeping a log to notice patterns of how Michael feels and what he is touching, smelling, or eating helped his mother address this behavior. He needs to notice patterns of what he is doing when he is overwrought with emotion because as an empath he needs to see that sometimes those are someone else's feelings. Also, he needs to notice smells, textures and foods that make him feel sick.

Read the book "The Impossible Child" By Doris Rapp. This book explains how food and chemicals can change personalities by common exposures found in the classroom. If you only deal with the chemicals at home but not at school his entire personality could change at school because of the chemicals around him.

The kid who is chemically sensitive may be a gift to other family members. Other family members may be sensitive to chemicals as well and when you have someone like Michael in the family everyone starts to read the labels and know what they are consuming. A brother or sister who has asthma suddenly can improve because the whole family changes what type of soap or laundry detergent they use.

Michael was not being rude or unfriendly or lacking empathy. Kids labeled as emotionally sensitive, who cry because others cry is not necessarily something that is a deficit. Empaths make great teachers, therapists, nurses or anything or even sales persons. Knowing another person's emotions gives you a distinct advantage because you are a built in lie detector. However, you can be labeled as oversensitive or a cry baby. Learn how to ground yourself and for an empath to recharge they need to be alone. People's energy will drain them and they prefer solitude or they have no energy left to do even the basic task. Read Empowered by Empathy by Rose Rosetree, and learn how even your unspoken emotions affect your child. This child will not watch violent television or movies and prefer solitude.

SARAH: The Burn Patient

Sarah's skin looked like it had burned, covered with tiny blisters. Some blisters were small and some were as a big as a centimeter and they covered her neck, scalp, back, knees and face. She had red marks on her legs from scratching and she squirmed in her seat because it felt uncomfortable to sit for long periods. Her doctor said to put cream on the skin for eczema, so she was using a product that contains oatmeal. This seemed to make her condition worse. No matter what she tried or skin ointment she used nothing seemed to work. Also, the flame retardant clothing her mother bought for her contained formaldehyde and it made her itch as well. Sarah preferred to wear the same red tee shirt every day because it was made of cotton and it did not have an itchy tag. She didn't even particularly like this tee shirt but it was the only one made of natural fibers. Sarah was a screamer and a scratcher because the pain, itchy, burning feeling would not go away.

Sarah had trouble sitting on swings because she preferred to put her belly on the swing and spin that made her feel slightly better. She was always looking at the floor, walking and pacing like she was about to vomit any minute. Sometimes she did. She was a champion at projectile vomiting because if there was a record for the biggest mess you make when you threw up Sarah surely hit the world record. She paced in circles, trying to get rid of the alien pain inside her. She sat curled up in a ball in constant tears as it felt as though her stomach was constricted as if someone put a corset on her that was way too tight and after every bite she would pace around the room. "make it stop" she thought to herself. What came out of her mouth however was pure screams of terror and vomit that would hit the opposite wall. School was a nightmare when they made her sit still because this was not possible especially after eating the school lunch. After lunch, she was in so much pain like a piano had fallen on her abdomen. Her tiny little protruding belly burst out of her skinny little body.

The itchy burning feeling was on her skin everywhere and she didn't like things touching her skin. She didn't like a casual hand on her shoulder and most definitely she did not like hugs. She would not use finger paint, or glue or play dough or anything that she had to touch with her hands because it just burned even more. She held her hands out like she was a surgeon ready for her next heart patient, avoiding all contact because it burned. Her mother was distraught and felt distant from Sarah because Sarah refused to let her mother hug her. Over many years, she had been to a pediatrician and a dermatologist who just told her to apply cream and said it was dermatitis but every cream she tried didn't work. In a feeble attempt to get Sarah to use the play dough, her mother gave her some plastic forks that she could cut or poke holes in the play dough to get nearer to being able to touch it. Sarah put all forty forks in the blob of play dough but still she would not touch it with her hands.

Sarah craved her mother and her sweet smell but when anything touched her skin the intense itchiness was overpowering. Sarah's mother thought Sarah had no feelings toward her because Sarah would not hug her mom. The closest thing to affection that Sarah could attempt was to lean on her mother like her mother was a comfortable place to sit next to but her mother was not allowed to touch. Her mother could see that Sarah really wanted to be around her mother but not touching and her mother had tried simply everything to help the eczema that was always on Sarah's skin. Anytime her mother touched Sarah, she would wince as if in pain.

Therapists had worked with Sarah to stand closer to other people when she talked to them or and they would use various media on the hands that were messy like painting and clay to help her learn how to get dirty. Sarah could eventually learn how to touch them with her hands but they still itched and burned and she still didn't like it. Sarah was three years old and was only slightly verbal but didn't have a phrase for itchy. She would say "no touch" when she could not bear the activity for that day.

Mostly Sarah spoke in two word phrases. She didn't know a word for itchy, scratch, burn, or hurt. She couldn't tell her mother that anything was wrong. Her little mind had figured out that her brain didn't function well or that she would forget simple things and get lost if she ate bread. Sarah's mother thought she was being rude and uncooperative when Sarah simply refused to eat the sandwiches that her mother had worked hard to make. Sarah knew something changed when she ate sandwiches and therefore refused to eat them. Her little mind was exploring what foods made her itch so that sometimes she ate and sometimes she didn't, but she had figured out that bread made her feel funny.

Sarah's mother thought she was just a picky eater and couldn't understand why she wouldn't touch the bread of her sandwich. She wouldn't eat the muffins and cookies that the other kids ate. She didn't even want her own birthday cake. She was skinny and labeled as "failure to thrive" because she was so short for her age and so tiny. Sarah's doctors never said the words autism because she was so young and instead, the doctor said she was developmentally delayed and thought that the reason she was not growing was because she wasn't eating. This was only partly true. It mattered a great deal what she was eating and she was going to need a drastic change to her diet to be well.

Sarah's mother had heard of people going gluten free and she decided to try it. As her mother was trying the new gluten free foods, Sarah didn't care for them at first because she did not know there was a difference in the new bread she was eating; she only knew that all bread made her sick. The rice cereal was a bit bland and she didn't like to eat very many vegetables. So, the beginning of trying out this diet, Sarah's mother had to improvise just to get her to eat anything. She didn't go completely gluten free at first because she needed to find things that Sarah liked. Her mother made an occasional mistake fixing Sarah something that she thought was gluten free only to find out later that it wasn't. She found out that the lotion had oatmeal in it and was causing the rash because it had gluten in it.

An interesting pattern emerged that when Sarah ate something with gluten in it the rashes returned and her skin completely cleared when she was 100% gluten free. Sarah's eczema was Dermatitis Herpetiformis, or a skin rash from eating gluten. Sarah went 100% gluten free and remains that way and if she eats anything or touches anything with gluten, her rash returns. But without it, she is happy and smiling and hugs her mother. She is social and talkative and willing and able to learn. She is growing like a weed but still should catch up to her peers. She can't understand why the teachers would give out cookies that would make her itch even if it is for Valentine's Day. Why would you eat something that makes you sick at a party? Everyone likes the new-found confidence and calm in Sarah and her skin looks beautiful.

Tools for Sarah's family

Because Sarah has Dermatitis Herpetiformis, a rash associated with gluten, a small infraction would be more easily noticeable than someone else with a gluten intolerance. Sarah is an extreme case of celiac with the rash that very few know about. She needs to use separate pans, even ovens, and can't even cook her foods in the same oils that had something cooked with gluten which would make eating in a restaurant very hard. Her food had to be made from scratch and completely 100% gluten free or her rash would return.

Soaps, lotions, medicines can have gluten and she should keep a watchful eye for hidden traces of gluten in all aspects of her life at home and at school. It's not always about how natural it is it's how your body reacts.

Sarah was not being rude or unfriendly or lacking empathy. Everything that touched her skin hurt, itched or burned and made her skin sensitive. She had to find the source to figure out the cause of the pain and correct it which for her was the gluten.

Sarah may need to make sense of all the gluten free things she can't have. It can make her feel like an outcast. People around her, though meaning well, tend to celebrate every holiday with food that she can't have and the deprivation could feel overwhelming. Help her find ways to celebrate without it being centered around food so that she doesn't always feel left out. People sometimes give therapy to kids like Sarah because they feel left out but if you are gluten free you ARE left out. Find ways to let her feel included instead of just dealing with her feelings. Read The Grain Brain by David Perlmutter.

Advice for Parents of Sensitive Children

Common Reasons Your Child Might be Sensitive
A child with mercury in their system can experience all their senses heightened. Everything is louder, brighter, smells stronger, taste stronger and can't hurt to touch. If the child has had a flu shot or has had dental amalgams, he should be checked for the mercury level. Read Vaccine Epidemic by Louise Habakus and Mary Holland, and Age of Autism by Dan Olmsted and Mark Blaxill.
Some kids are pain sensitive and a withdrawal from touch is because the touch is painful. What is on their skin or touching it that would cause pain? Figuring out what is causing the pain is difficult in a nonverbal child but some of the first words they use whether they communicate via an iPad, typing, or speaking they need to learn words for ouch, hurt, pain, itch, scratch and burns.
Kids labeled as emotionally sensitive, who cry because others cry, are not behaving in a way that is necessarily a deficit. Empaths make great teachers, therapists, nurses or anything or even sales persons.
Many of our kids react to gluten but extreme rashes are uncommon. Because many of our kids have a "leaky gut" and the gluten goes to the brain gives them a high feeling, and what they are doing is mostly a reaction to the gluteomorphin in their brain. Many parents make the mistake of just going gluten free, but choose lactose free milk, when the lactose is not the problem. Lactose is milk fat. The problem is the casein or the milk protein. If your child has a problem with gluten, try removing the casein from the diet not the lactose.

Possible Medical Reasons Your Child Might be Sensitive
Lyme (it might be diagnosed as fibromyalgia or MS but may be Lyme)
Mercury
Chemicals
Candida (can also cause a rash)
Aluminum
PANDAS also can have a rash like scarlet fever.
Various other shedding from vaccines cause reactions.
Celiac causes a rash as well.
Empathic

The Learning-Disabled Child

DOUGLAS: Obsessed with Letters and Numbers

Some parents of three year olds will put their kids in time out with a timer to let them know how long they are supposed to sit. Douglas loved timers and counted down excitedly with the timer like he was an astronaut getting ready for liftoff. "Ten, Nine, Eight, Seven, Six, Five, Four, Three, Two, One." By the time he got to one he was squealing running in circles with his hands on his ears. He was so excited he would burst! His mother not only had to get rid of the timer during time out but cover up all the clocks he could see because he was just as excited to count on the clock until it was time to get up. Douglas could never sit if there was a countdown somewhere. That was way too much fun!

Douglas was not a spy but he did speak a secret code. If you watched the shows that Douglas watched and saw the movies that he saw then sometimes the phrases that seemed to be out of context, made perfect sense. He created his own phrases to explain himself and his surroundings that he was quoting verbatim from what television and movies but he picked them particularly for their content and relevance. He could not explain what things were called. He could not answer questions unless you could speak in his code. One of these phrases was "Eight Hundred Dollars." To the teacher or friend that didn't understand Douglas they might have thought he was obsessed with money. an exact amount of eight hundred dollars. Douglas said this at exactly 7:30 every evening when *Wheel of Fortune* was on television.

He would say "Eight Hundred Dollars! I want eight hundred dollars!!" which meant he wanted to watch *Wheel of Fortune* his favorite show because it had letters and numbers. The first time he saw the show, this is the number they spun on the wheel, so to him the show was called "Eight Hundred Dollars." Though he could not always explain himself or answer a question, when he was watching Wheel of Fortune he did sometimes guess correctly the clues on the show.

Another way that Douglas communicated was creating his own code for car. He didn't know what a car was and didn't have a word for car but he did notice license plates. He not only noticed but he remembered his mother's license plate and he could find her car anywhere at any time. He would say "XYQ1975" when he wanted to go somewhere. This was the license plate on his mother's car. "XYQ1975" was his word for car. He would say "XYQ1975" and take her hand and go right to it. She never had to worry about losing her car in the parking lot. She would say, "Douglas, where is XYQ1975?" She had to ask several times and make sure he was looking at her to give him time to respond.

When he understood, he would grab her by the elbow and run exactly to her car no matter where it was or how much traffic was in the parking lot. She had to make sure there was no traffic and that he was aware of the other cars so he wouldn't get run over but at least she knew where he was going and that once he found her car, he would wait for her. He grabbed her and pulled her directly to the car ignoring cars, stop signs and other pedestrians but he always found the car right away and stood in front of the license plate running in circle excited that he had found it. She needed to teach him to take his time, slow down and watch for oncoming traffic. His running was not random; it had a purpose and a finish line. If he made it there safely, he had won. Timing to get there was everything and he had to win the race.

Douglas's obsession for timing carried over to dates, calendars and clocks. If his mother wanted him to do something at a certain time, he wanted to do it at exactly that time and not one more second. His code was that he would say. "Bed at seven oh oh" which meant that he wanted to go to bed at 7:00. He meant at seven o'clock exactly not 6:59 or 7:01. He was angry that the microwave clock and the stove clock were not synchronized and both did not change to 7:00 at the same second. He held his ears and screamed until they both displayed the same time. Calendars created similar obsessive behavior.

If he went to bed on January 31 and when he woke up at three in the morning, he knew it was February, and would scream and point at the calendar because it had not been changed to February at exactly midnight. His mother spent a lot of time synchronizing clocks, calendars and the timing of everything she did to avoid his meltdowns that the timing of his activities in his mind was wrong. However, one could also admire that he could tell time, he knew the days of the week, months of the year and he could count change. His young mind was brilliant and advanced but also exhausting.

This ability to concentrate on numbers and letters also translated to amazing math ability. When Douglas was three years old, his grandpa looked in his wallet and said he had seventy-eight dollars when he had bought forty-five dollars' worth of gas. Douglas sat in the car and squealed, and meant to say thirty-three but since he couldn't say his TH or R sounds it came out "Fahty fee" He knew seventy-eight minus forty-five was thirty-three.

Douglas loved Karaoke. He knew the words to lots of songs, and if his mom gave him the lyrics written down he could read them. But with Karaoke the words were highlighted as they were sung on the machine, and he not only heard the word but could see it at the same time. It helped him to process what he saw to match what he heard. Sometimes kids on the spectrum have a delay, so Karaoke was helpful *and* fun.

Douglas loved to watch television and movies as well with subtitles because again he could see what was said and hear it and there was a picture to visualize what the words meant. He had difficulty with slang and metaphors because he took them literally. If his mother said it was raining cats and dogs, Douglas would look up to the sky and giggle waiting for the cats and dogs to come. Douglas had also picked up a phrase that he did not quite understand. It said "You rock!" Annie explained to him that this meant I love you. Douglas would collect special rocks and give them to people he liked. His mother had a collection of special rocks.

Douglas loved rules because there were specific directions written down that he could follow. He read the road signs which were the rules of the road, the playground rules, even the directions to the games his Mom wanted him to play. If the directions said the game for age three and up. He would not play because he was four years old and he thought he was too old to play because he understood that this meant only three-year old could play. This cumbersome rule kept him from enjoying board games because there were days that he would rather read the rules of the game rather than play, or not play at all if they were not followed to his specifications exactly.

Douglas's mom thought she could use his word obsession and his love of rules to her advantage but she had to get him to have better comprehension so that he could improve communication and start naming actual objects correctly instead of making up his own names for things. She knew if things had labels he would go right to it and read the words. She put labels on the couch, chair, and table. Douglas would point to the sign that said couch and say "couch". The trick was for him to understand that the object was a couch not just to point to the word. He also had difficulty with the idea that sometimes there was more than one word for the same thing. If someone called the couch a sofa it would confuse him. It could only be a couch. While therapists used pictures with most kids to get them to expand their vocabulary, they did not use words. Though his mother explained this to them, one of them said "but we won't do that because Douglas is too young to learn how to read."

Douglas knew advanced words and was an expert and decoding words he had never seen before. If the therapist used pictures to explain things this slowed down his learning process because it was not how he learned and remembered. Douglas needed to connect the word to the object when in school we are taught to connect the object to the word. One could assume that he could already read the word but he may not understand what it meant. When his mother spelled drink, and held up a glass this was her way of showing him how to connect the word drink to the glass. Then the next time he was thirsty, he had to say drink to show he knew the meaning.

Douglas's mom Annie noticed that when Grandpa was wearing a baseball cap with an A on it, Douglas would sit on his lap and look directly at the hat. If Grandpa wore a t-shirt with words on it Douglas would look at that as well. He didn't look at Grandpa's face or even say Grandpa or acknowledge who he was, but if Grandpa wore anything with writing on it, Douglas willingly sat on Grandpa's lap.

His mother used the same idea to label objects as to label people. She took a post-it note and wrote "mommy" on it and put it on her face, between her eyes. Douglas looked right at it, right between her eyes and said "mommy." He had never called her Mommy before or looked into her eyes either. He screamed and cried looking into people's eyes but somehow focuses on the words which to him were much easier to understand and much less scary.

What if you were an American who went on a tour of Spain but only knew a little Spanish? Douglas's own phrases were like his first language. When he had to navigate through the world and learn actual names of things those were like learning another language. For him to learn more quickly, he needed teachers and therapists had to see the world and understand it the way he did. Just like the tourist who didn't understand the language in Spain, when someone did not understand what he said instead of rephrasing or trying to explain what he meant, Douglas screamed and spoke louder as if the reason people didn't understand was because he was not loud enough not because their way of speaking felt foreign to him.

One of his teachers was brilliant and used software that had the word "pop" and it popped and the word "squeeze" would squeeze. She was showing them words that did the action that it said and it was very helpful to teach him verbs. Douglas needed a way to be able to explain words that were not all nouns to be able to speak in full sentences.

Douglas had his own version of imaginary play. He counted the matchbox cars and separated the ones with numbers on the sides and the plain ones without numbers. He picked up the one with the number two and said Two. His eyes lit up with excitement. The cars with numbers or letters again were clearly his favorite. It might look like he was counting the cars but if you looked closer he was randomly counting and the number of actual cars was not important. Sometimes Douglas counted to himself to calm down or ran in circles and flapped his hands when he was excited again he was counting but this time it was a countdown.

Since Annie couldn't label pain or teach Douglas how to recognize it she needed to find a better way to explain it. She pointed to his stuffed bear's paw and said. "Ouch" and put a band aid on that same place. She wrote Ouch on the band-aid. The next time Douglas fell, Annie put a band-aid on his cut and

Douglas suddenly said, "Ouch". For kids on the spectrum being able to tell someone you are hurt is extremely important.

Annie made up a game. The game was called "treasure." Douglas knew the word *desk* and the word *ball* and he knew their meaning but the game was to see if he knew under, over, or between. She wrote "The ball is under the desk." If Douglas could find the ball he understood the sentence.

Douglas's therapists used these methods to teach him how to have conversations by writing down short scripts and social stories to tell him to what to say in certain circumstances. Then the therapists would put him with other kids to facilitate those circumstances and give him practice having those conversations with other children. If the other kid said something different, he would be confused because they did not follow the script. This would help him maintain conversations to be able to answer and ask questions.

Douglas confused people because he was brilliant, but still on the spectrum. Because he didn't understand questions all the time, people had to ask him many times and give him a chance to think about a response. Teachers thought he was learning disabled, but when they checked his reading levels, he was several grades higher than his peers on sight-reading, but slower in comprehension. Therefore, when he was told to read the books on his grade level, he resisted because he was bored.

His math skills were also quite advanced but he couldn't explain his thinking. It was almost like words were his first language and writing was his second. So even though he could spell beautifully he was slow writing it all down. What he did write down was not nearly as creative as the story that was in his head because his thoughts were so quick. Douglas was Hyperlexic and Twice Exceptional, meaning he was advanced on some skills and behind in others.

Tools for Douglas's Family

Hyperlexia is a condition in which kids can read very early but sometimes have developmental challenges around reading. There is much debate as to whether it is considered autism or just sometimes misdiagnosed. Scientific American puts it in subtypes and some of two of three of those subtypes are considered part of autism. My children had this ability and I use this story based on my own experience and what worked to help them with language, comprehension, and the strength to decode and spell a large variety of words.

Here are some tips I used to improve comprehension that are illustrated in this story.

Watch movies and TV with subtitles to connect what they hear with the words they see.

Karaoke to learn the same thing with music

Labeling objects around the house to connect the word to the object.

Software or other tools to improve comprehension for adjectives and verbs. We did flashcards for sight words.

Give your child the correct words to use by sometimes spelling it for him and showing him the word then using it to ask for what he wants. "I want a drink."

Social stories for certain situations your child might have difficulty so he can think about the activity and plan what to say ahead of time and then offer verbal coaching if needed.

Any rules you want your child to follow or a schedule, write it down.

ABA and PECS does not address kids that are Hyperlexic. PECS stands for Picture Exchange Communication System unless the pictures have words underneath. There are some programs that do but not all. Anything such as flash cards with words and pictures would help a child connect the words to the objects.

I strongly recommend with all kids not to downgrade, or ignore any gift your child has. Schools tend to focus on the weaknesses. The ideas listed here are things I did with my kids to help give them a vocabulary.

Read When Babies Read: A Practical Guide to Helping Children with Hyperlexia, Asperger's And High Functioning Autism by Audra Jensen

WILLIAM: The Fumbling Child

William was always squinting. He was terrible at sports and when his mom signed him up for Soccer it was a total disaster because he didn't see the ball until it literally hit him in the head. Any sport he tried he didn't see any balls coming at him. He was labeled as uncoordinated, with poor motor planning and hypotonic or weak muscle tone.

Though he could read very well, the chapter books were hard. He didn't just a skip a few words; he skipped entire lines and paragraphs of text, and small words like *a* and *the*. When the teacher told him to look at the smart board to read something from a distance, he could see it but then he had to look down as his paper and didn't know what he was supposed to be doing because he had lost his place. While he was trying to figure out what everyone was doing and where in the book they were, they had moved on and he was further lost. Then looking back up at the teacher he was further lost. As his day progressed and other kids moved effortlessly from the board the desk and back the board, each time there was a shift, Douglas was a little more lost. He lost his place, lost his book and had no idea what he was supposed to be doing.

William had figured out some tricks to fix this but his teacher told him to stop because she didn't understand why they were helping. As he was reading he used his finger, a bookmark or a ruler to mark his place. When he did math, his errors were almost always because the numbers were not lined up correctly so he drew lines to fix it. His teacher told him that was slowing him down and he should be able to line up the numbers on his own but he couldn't. This misunderstanding caused him to make more errors because he could not line up the numbers to add correctly. It took him an extensive period of time to check and recheck and check again. He understood the math and all the concepts but the teacher saw simple clerical mistakes and said he wasn't checking his work.

William lost his way in other areas too. When he climbed the ladder to the slide, his foot would miss the step and he would stumble. Sometimes when he walked down the hall, he said he felt disoriented and dizzy and insisted that he hold onto the wall for support. When he sat in a chair he had to touch around the chair to make sure it was where he thought it would be or he would sit at an angle and fall off. Sometimes when he put his tray down at lunch he had to check to make sure it was fully on the table because sometimes it was only partly on the table and it only took a misplaced elbow to dump his food on the floor. He made messes when he ate and was constantly dropping his food and getting drips on his clothing. He couldn't even make it to his mouth without spilling. He was called a klutz by his own family, and teased for his inability to play sports and constantly making messes.

When he was reading for a long time, he rubbed his eyes and took very long blinks. He yawned, stretched, and laid his head on his desk. He starred out the window. His eyes felt like he had poked needles in them and they stung. When he looked at the words they seemed to float in space right off the page. He would blink and stare and try to focus but the words would still move around. When the ball came at him he felt blinded for a second and he felt attacked by a hidden tiger. Each sport he played he was completely blindsided by where the ball would be because he was hit all the time so he would duck and cover to protect his head as if an earthquake was about to hit.

He had a reading tutor, a writing tutor and a math tutor to help with his deficits. The words floated in midair when he looked at them and when he squinted or rubbed his eyes or blinked a long time that did not help at all. He was marked off for skipping words when he was reading out loud so his reading level was a grade lower than it should be and he was given books that were way too easy for him. When he had to write a story, he had the ideas and he was motivated but the time it took to form the letters on the paper took effort and the words were not written on the line but at an upward slope. The effort it took to write made writing so slow that by the time he got to the next sentence he had forgotten what he wanted to write about so there was a huge gap between the words he was going to write in his head and the ones that were on the paper.

His teacher gave him helper worksheets which had space to put character, setting or plot in an outline format to recall later. This helped but it didn't improve the time it took for him to write down what he wanted to say. He had a lot of incompletes and didn't finish his work. He wished his teachers would let him do his work on a computer because it was a lot less tiring and the writing was so much clearer.

Sometimes words switched places when he read. Sometimes he reread the same paragraph over and over. The small print was microscopic and the large print was too simplistic and easy for him. He needed to read chapter books with large print.

His mom took him to the eye doctor. When the doctor shined, a light left to right in front of his eyes, he had to move his whole head instead of just his eyes to follow. Sometimes his eyes would shift backwards a little or his right eye would straight ahead and his left eye would look off in a distance. He needed to focus both eyes on the same object at the same time and be able to follow an object placed in front of him with only his eyes not his whole head. His eye doctor recommended vision therapy.

Vision therapy was a lot of activity involving catching a ball beginning with a large playground ball and working to towards a small bouncing ball for him to track with his eyes. Other activities involved looking at similar letters like b, d, p, and q and he would point to each letter with a metronome timer.

Or he had to look at the first and last letter of each line of a book so that he would practice not losing his place where he was reading. He played a lot of ball and sports activities to keep track of catching the ball and seeing it when it came to him. He also wore special glasses called Prism glasses that magnified the words in the center to give him one place to focus. The therapist told him to walk with a flashlight pointing at a balance beam in front of him to help him to focus and see where he was walking both trying this forwards and backwards this would keep him from feeling disoriented and to watch where he was going with both eyes at the same time. He had a year of intense therapy to improve his tracking and focus on his eyes and to continue to wear the prism glasses.

After a year, the therapist retested him and amazingly he quadrupled what he could write in the same timeframe that he had before the test. When he started, he could not catch a large playground ball but now he could catch a small bouncy ball. He could climb a rock wall and even skateboard. The most important thing that he gained was that he no longer needed the reading, writing or math tutors because his grades went up in every subject across the board because he was finally learning at his appropriate grade level. He was in third grade now reading at a sixth-grade level. Now not only was he writing beautifully and distinctly but his teacher used his writing as an example to show the other kids how to write and he even started some advanced math. Physical Education was something that he had detested before because he kept getting hit with a ball but now he enjoyed it and asked his mom to play soccer with him. Something as simple as a vision therapy can completely change how William saw the world and moved through it. Since he stopped falling and could catch a ball he could play sports, which began to change how others saw William.

Tools for William's Family

Answer these questions to find out if your child needs vision therapy.

- Can your child track a ball?
- When your child is reading, does she skip whole lines or paragraphs instead of specific words?
- Does your child sit on the chair and miss or feel around and touch the chair before she sits down?
- Can your child climb a ladder or the stairs? Does he have to touch the rungs of the ladder or touch the stairs before climbing?
- Does your child walk down the hall touching the wall to hold her balance?
- Does your child fall down a lot?

William could not track a ball or follow along reading with his classmates because the words seem to float around the page. He could not see the transition between reading close up and far away and something as simple as Prism glasses can fix it.

One clue to see if a child has a tracking problem is to see if he can follow a flashlight moving in front of his face by only moving his eyes. William had to move his whole head because this was too difficult.

Read the book Seeing Through New Eyes Changing the Lives of Children with Autism, Asperger's and other Developmental Disabilities Through Vision Therapy by Melvin Kaplan.

Advice To Parents with Learning-Disabled Kids

Commonly Overlooked Causes of Learning Disabilities

Can your child hear or see properly? Is there anything that is preventing this? Any child with a learning disability should be checked including for tracking or vision difficulties. How do you know?

Does your child squint, rub his eyes, or blink slowly or too often?

Does your child have a good sense of balance or inner ear?

Does your child have a lot of ear infections, or fluid in the ear? Do they push, pull or tug on the ears? Fluid in the ear sounds like everything is under water and difficult to process language. Clean the ears of fluid, wax or reduce inflammation may improve attention. The child doesn't pay attention because he can't hear you and because he can't speak he can't tell you.

Do the eyes get red, blotchy, inflamed? Do they get pink eye or allergies of the eye?

Can your child catch a ball?

Does your child look at you when you say his name?

Can he communicate his needs by pointing, gesturing or any other communication with pictures or words?

Does your child have dysgraphia because of pain? Sometimes kids can't tell you what hurts unless you ask. If your child can't speak then look for signs of inflammation, or rubbing their hands or parts of the body that are physically inflamed that might keep them from writing to their ability.

Consider using computers, or iPads or other devices to encourage communication. If the child can't speak and can't write things down, he may be able to use a keyboard if given enough time to write down their thoughts. An iPad with the proper application for communication can be his lifeline to connect to the world. A computer can also help him to write stories if writing by hand is too difficult. Consider this for a child with poor writing skills or to give him reading material on a Kindle and increase the font size for a kid with poor eyesight.

There is sometimes a gap between what the child hears and watching the person's lips move as if he is watching a movie with the picture not linked with the sound. That's why karaoke and subtitles might be very beneficial.

Don't ignore a gift like a child who can read at very young age. Hyperlexia can be great way to give language by labeling objects, using flash cards, descriptions of textures and colors using words and things that use a picture or a description along with a word that they already know by sight reading but may not know the meaning. Give them the meaning and you give them a vocabulary.

Don't allow your kid if he wants to use different words for things. For a proper communication to develop between peers he needs to learn the proper words for things and allowing him to use the proper words for things will help his expressive language. Give him the time and space as the correct words are a second language and his made-up word is a foreign language. In other words, it may take time for him to understand or there is a language barrier until he begins to think about objects using the correct words for things. You may have to use different phrases or give him a different context to help him to learn what you are asking.

Even neurotypical children have difficulty with slang and metaphors at a young age. So, if your child has difficulty teach him a slang word or phrase of the day and have a reward system for using it correctly. These take time. Think about when and where you use these phrases so that he is not embarrassed in front of people when he takes something too literal.

Social stories can be very helpful to learn how to have conversations and how to answer who what when where and why or open ended questions. You can role play and help him plan the types of questions people might ask and how to answer even if he uses a computer or iPad to do it.

The Hyper Child
ANDREW: The Squirmy Kid

Andrew knew how to do one thing and that was run. He knew how to run away and never noticed that this was a busy highway and he could be run over. He would run out on the street unaware of traffic and not look both ways. Andrew sometimes would hit himself on the arms and legs because it felt like there were tiny army ants crawling all over his body. Andrew could never sit still because his bottom was painful and itchy. Instead, Andrew squirmed at his desk, sat sideways and tried moving around in his seat to get comfortable but he did not get up from his seat, he just sat and move around because when he stood up he had pressure on his joints in his legs and feet hurt. They hurt less when he sat down but he still had to constantly shift in his chair.

Andrew had constipation and diarrhea. He had anxiety and stress about the world in general and he would run to escape. Little things overwhelmed him and he shut out the world by covering his ears when the world seemed too much. When this wasn't good enough, he would escape by walking out of the room.

Andrew's mother had too many calls from the school to count. They could not stop him from swatting his arms and legs as if he was covered in flies. They gave him gloves to stop scratching. The teachers couldn't keep up with him and he had an aide who had to constantly run after him.

One thing that Andrew could do well and very quickly was run. He could out run everyone in PE easily and still have energy to spare. He was trying to run away from everyone and everything without a plan or a care. Andrew thought that if he ran far enough, maybe his arms wouldn't feel so prickly and itchy. Even when he stopped running, he couldn't stop scratching.

Andrew's mother had finally decided that public school was not a good fit because he was constant squirming and then running into danger. He had to wear a bracelet to track him and figure out where he would go. Eventually he grew tired and would walk and they would find him somewhere in the neighborhood, sitting down because he was too tired to walk. Eventually his mother decided to home school because she literally could not keep up with him. No wonder he couldn't concentrate. Andrew always felt like he needed to poop, but he just couldn't and what would come out looked like blood mixed with something found in your tissue after blowing your nose. Andrew could never seem to go to the bathroom but not for lack of trying. When he could finally go, a baseball size ball would come out.

Andrew had parasites. His symptoms of anxiety, gastrointestinal and his feeling of ants on his body, and painful joints were all his symptoms even though many people with parasites have no symptoms at all. He was squirming in his seat, this was his way of relieving that itch, and swatting himself was trying to stop the feeling of ants crawling on him. His doctor did a stool analysis and found the parasites he had and the protocol that was needed to fix it. [245,246]

As the doctor treated his gut, she used a protocol from Hulda Clark which used black walnut, wormwood and cloves. [247] Andrew had to defecate more often, and when he did, his mannerisms had changed because his intestines were becoming healthy He became less nervous over all and less things bothered him.

He had even let his mother hug him and read him a bedtime story. For him to sit still through a whole story was a miracle. He liked to run now for fun and now he enjoyed his P.E. classes because he usually was ahead of his peers. Running needed to be included as part of his day to cope with daily stress. But also to be taught are skills that involved sitting as well.

Tools for Andrew and his family
Andrew used to run as an escape and to add to that he was very fast. His energy needed to be channeled to learn when and where it was okay to run and not to literally run away from things that bothered him. This was his coping strategy and he needed better ways to deal with things that were uncomfortable both physically, or things causing stress. He had to learn other ways to deal with stress besides running.
Andrew's bottom itched, he had joint pain, and gastrointestinal upset were his symptoms of parasites. Though many people with parasites have no symptoms, these were his.

BENJAMIN: The Screamer

Benjamin's feet hurt. His legs felt like they were burning. Hot searing pain on his legs, ankles and calves to his knees. Benjamin walked across the floor like he was walking on hot coals. He walked on his toes and they barely touched the ground. He walked with short quick little steps and never ever put his heels down because that's where the fire felt like it must be. He would try to swat out the fire with his hands and he would hit his legs repeatedly and sometimes his legs would twitch during the day and in the middle of the night. The feeling of being on fire would keep him awake and he couldn't sleep at all. He could scream and he could cry but he could not tell anyone that his feet felt like burning from the inside out. He could not speak and he was restless because he so desperately wanted to tell someone about the fiery burning sensation he was feeling in his legs. He even tried to run from the fire. He ran everywhere to escape from the pain, but the fire followed him wherever he went. His legs weren't really on fire but they felt insanely hot and painful.

Benjamin refused to wear shoes and always took them off. Shoes seem to make the burning worse and when he had to wear them he kicked them off. He ran away when he could because the pain was here and he had to be somewhere else. It was like the inside of his body was on fire but the outside didn't have a scratch. The myelin sheath that surrounds the nerves in his legs were very damaged and this burning sensation was a result of his nervous system on overdrive. He hated being hugged or touched in anyway because the slightest touch felt like a blowtorch. His clothes felt like sandpaper and everything that was anywhere near his skin hurt. He would not touch anything or let anyone touch him because his nerves were like stripped wires and sensitive to everything.

Benjamin and his Grandma were trying to go on a low sugar diet and so every sweetener they ate had aspartame or the brand name Equal which his grandma thought was better. Aspartame in his milk, cereal, yogurt, Coke, and cookies. They ate everything with aspartame and their aches and pains only grew worse. Benjamin and his Grandma ate a lot of things with artificial colors and had no idea that it was a problem because his Grandma never looked at the ingredients too carefully.

Benjamin had to be homeschooled because his need to run was overwhelming and his way of coping from the pain. His grandmother couldn't understand why he was screaming for no reason and waking all the old ladies that lived near her house. She couldn't cope with him swatting his legs and didn't know how to deal with it. She had fibromyalgia and her legs felt like a thousand pins on them and she just didn't want anyone touching her either she just felt old and frail and in pain. Both Benjamin and Grandma had nerve damage in their legs.

Grandma could tell someone what was wrong and Benjamin couldn't. But their causes were similar.

Tools for Benjamin and his family
Remove all Aspartame sometimes listed as Aspartic Acid or Phenylalanine in the ingredients. Watch a movie called *Sweet Poison* and see how aspartame can harm your health. It can cause symptoms like fibromyalgia.
Read the story about Lisa Marks Smith, who had nerve damage after a flu shot.
Pay attention to how others in the family are feeling. Both Benjamin and his grandma had nerve damage. Grandma rubs her feet in pain and Benjamin hits himself in the leg. Even when kids can't talk they can still tell you in their own way that they are in pain.

Common Reasons for Hyperactivity
Pain
On overdrive because of lack of sleep.
Gut problems like Candida
Find out what he is running to or from?
Why is he climbing and does he have a goal to get there? Cookies?
Check for allergies.
Some kids are labeled hyper in school because the work is too easy or too hard. They are bored.

Possible Medical Reasons for Hyperactivity

Lyme
Candida
Parasites
Celiac or opiate addiction to food
Lead
Mercury
Medications
Allergies
Artificial colors and sugars

The Exhausted Child
JUSTIN: Tired and Slow

Justin walked like a gorilla as if his arms were way too long. He slumped over and dragged his feet everywhere he went. He held his pencil in a tight-fisted grip as if he was going to stab the paper and frequently ripped holes as he pressed down too hard. He told his mom "I'm an old man." And he walked as though he was. His hands were cramped and felt arthritic like an old man. There was pain in the knuckles and they were inflamed and swollen. His neck sometimes was sore and painful as well as if he could not turn his head. His knees were raw and usually large for the rest of his frail thin legs. His feet hurt when he walked and he would much prefer to sit down and give them a break.

Justin could talk but much of what came out of his mouth was a complaint about everything. He complained the most about his physical education class because it involved running. Running the track in PE was like trying to run a marathon with both your legs broken. His legs were not broken but they felt like they would snap any second.

Most days, Justin was so tired he couldn't stand up and was constantly angry at anyone who made him do any work because it was all just too much. His hands hurt and he couldn't make them write what was in his head even when he tried hard. He couldn't grip the pencil to make words. He couldn't keep the words in his head long enough to write them down. He forgot his homework, he misplaced his backpack, and he was always late for school searching for his shoes. He had some support to help him organize and some days he could remember everything. The next day, he would forget. His tests showed either an A or an F and nothing in between depending whether he had eaten gluten or not. His worst class by far was physical education. It was more like torture for Justin. He tried to run but his legs just felt like lead. His whole body felt heavy as if he was an eighty-year-old man with fifty-pound weights on his leg. No matter what the temperature, he was freezing from the inside of his body, as if it had no central heating. Kids made fun of him for wearing big heavy sweatshirts when it was 85 degrees but that was the only way he could keep warm and Justin never ever felt warm.

He handed in the work he could manage to do but his teachers and his family thought he just wasn't trying and put him in extra classes to make him work even harder. Justin was failing his physical education classes because he could not run and he could barely walk. In his mind, he thought of all the great things he was going to do and what kind of job he wanted when he grew up, but he wasn't sure he had the stamina to be a teacher because they stood up all day long and that just looked exhausting. His mother said he was lazy because he would do some chores but not finish. He would sweep the dirt on the kitchen floor into a pile but sit down for ten minutes before he put it into the dustpan. He had the same trouble at school and sometimes didn't finish his tasks especially if they involved standing up for long periods. He didn't just want to sit down; he had to sit down because he felt his legs could no longer support him.

Justin was verbal and considered shy. He chose very carefully who and under what circumstances he would talk. He never raised his hand in class but he frequently knew the answers to the questions. If he did answer and he was wrong, and if anyone said anything or laughed, that was one class in which he would never say another word. He talked to the kids who sat around him but sometimes he just could not bring himself to speak. They gave him special pencil grips to hold the pencil firmer and extra work to encourage him to write more often because on a good day, he wrote beautifully. On a bad day, he wrote scribble. His teachers knew his ideas were well thought out because he could explain them but he couldn't write them down. His anger was at himself for not being able to make his hands write down his thoughts well enough to get a good grade in any of his classes. His anger was also directed at school where there was so much homework and it took all the energy he had to do anything. His anger reflected frustration, a stress level that he could never explain and he was tired of trying because no one listened. Justin pretended everything was fine until it just wasn't. Most of the time, Justin was good-natured but didn't talk very much. He was quiet and had a million thoughts racing in his mind about what he wanted to do that day but he was just too exhausted to do them. When he really could no longer just "tough it out" as his mother said, he would break down and quit. He would refuse to do homework or even anything in school.

Because Justin was so quiet at school they just said at first, he was shy and he was not living up to his potential. His parents took him to a therapist where he finally told them how sick and tired he felt, how he couldn't concentrate on anything and how he could not get anyone in school to understand how much he suffered. Other students who would talk to him thought he was smart but they didn't get too close because sometimes he would just scream at them for seemingly no reason. At his highest stress and frustration levels, he screamed, he bit, and he threw things. His pain was excruciating. Fatigue was washing over him like the ocean had knocked him over and he was too tired to move. His parents put him in tutoring classes to help him improve his memory but he still couldn't grasp why sometimes he could not remember names, dates or objects. He complained about being cold but thought why bother and would wear a gigantic winter coat no matter what the temperature. He told people he just liked this coat but the truth was he never felt warm.

Justin was diagnosed with selective mutism and hypotonia. He was behind his peers in large and small motor skills but technically not part of autism because under the right circumstances he could talk if he chose. He did need support in school to organize and finish his tasks with prompts. People did not want to talk to him because they said he complained too much so he just stopped talking. But the fact was, he had real things to complain about but they were overlooked by his doctors, teachers, and therapist.

Tools for Justin and His Family
Send a letter to the school to specify the child's medical conditions to show that the reason the child is tired is because of Lyme for example, not because he is lazy. Do not let the child fail a class because he is medically unable to complete it. Get accommodations to fit your situation and meet him at his level.
Justin was cold all the time and people could see that because he was always overdressed and wore heavy coats in the summer because he was hypothyroid which would make him very tired.
If he has complained to his mother and nothing in his situation has changed, he may not do it again. He needs to feel heard and respected for his "complaining" and to be given a break when needed.
Keep a food diary which also rates how he feels that day. He may notice a pattern of fatigue associated with certain foods. Some people can become exhausted after eating gluten and if they are eating it all the time they are constantly exhausted. The moment of clarity comes when you don't eat it and function better.
Lyme, Candida[248] and mitochondrial dysfunction are all good things to test for if you have the exhausted child because unless you test that's the only way to tell and the fatigue may be your only clue. Antibiotics and sugar can make this even worse. Antibiotics are a common treatment for Lyme.
Anger is expressed when exhaustion escalates to overworking and frustration. When medical issues are addressed and the child is less tired he will finish his tasks. This can take a long time depending on the issues. Therapy is more efficient and cheaper because you need less if you are not exhausted. Have you ever gone to work if you didn't sleep the night before? Did a coworker help you finish your tasks?

CALEB: The Snorer

Caleb walked off balance and he fell down all the time. He walked around dizzy and disoriented as if he was walking on a boat moving very fast. The floor felt unsteady and wobbly and he had to hold on to the wall for balance. He walked into furniture and into people as if he wasn't aware they were there until he bumped into them.

Caleb heard people talking in muffled voices as if he was under water, and their voices sounded distant. His ears felt like he was on a plane at a very high altitude and they were about to pop. He could faintly hear them say his name. "Caleb" his mother would say. He heard that. The rest was a muffle. Sometimes he really wanted his ears to pop and he would put his hands on his ears to try to relieve the pressure.

Caleb was so tired he would sleep in physical education class. The other kids would run over him and jump over him. Caleb didn't sleep very well and last night was no exception. He woke up at 11, 2, 4, and 5:00. He didn't know why he was so exhausted but sometimes he just had to let nature take over no matter where he was.

Caleb slept during the day in all the wrong places. He breathed loudly like he was asthmatic. Mold and pollen made his throat more inflamed than it already was and he would breathe even louder when he was outside running around. He had a constant hacking cough that would go away and come back several times and he had been on every antibiotic that ever existed because he was sick so often.

At night Caleb slept loudly like a leaf blower was in his room. He snored so loud that no one in the house could sleep. He took deep breaths and sometimes for a second or two he stopped breathing and then let in a big intake of air as if he was choking. When he stopped breathing it woke him up and he would toss and turn all over the bed. He went to bed with his head on the pillow and woke up with his feet where his head should be. He had squirmed so much that his feet and his head had switched places. He moved in fits and snored like a buzz saw all night and he had not slept well in years. He had constant sore throats, strep, bronchitis, ear infections, and colds. He was constantly sick and breathed through his mouth sticking out his tongue to give more space to breathe. Caleb had inflamed tonsils, and adenoids and constant ear infections. After one visit to the dentist, the dentist told Caleb's mother to take him to an Ear, Nose, and Throat Doctor at just three years old.

The ENT doctor told him he needed tubes in his ears and his tonsils, and adenoids out because of the snoring and all the times he was sick. Caleb didn't like the feeling of water in dripping in his ears but suddenly when people spoke to him they didn't sound like they were talking under water. They were crystal clear. Because they no longer sounded like gibberish he could respond.

In fact, as he started healing, he insisted that his mom give "medicine" to his stuffed Curious George and would insist that George had the same medical care he did. This was big news for Caleb because he had never really done any imaginary play before.

That night when his mother put Caleb to bed, he slept so quietly, she had to check to see if he was breathing. There was no snoring, no noises, and no rustling. He was completely asleep by 7:30 that night and stayed asleep until morning. For the first time, Caleb slept through the night!

After a few days of this, Caleb was suddenly hungry for everything and wanted to try the broccoli on his brother's plate and even said "broccoli". He was using new words. He was looking at the person's face, not always the eyes, but acknowledging that they were speaking to him. He was awake and alert during the day, and could sit at a table to learn more easily. He even hugged his mom.

Tools for Caleb's Family
When Caleb has told me, that he was walking, "it felt like water". He held onto the wall for balance. Later, we only learn that his vestibular function was not working properly. Physical, Occupational and Vision Therapy can improve balance and coordination
Mold, dust and other allergies and viruses can make the tonsils inflamed. If you can remove the allergens, you can prevent the stuffy nose and mouth breathing. Sometimes parents must be a detective.
The inflammation in his ears nose and throat was preventing proper drainage. If he were to take something like an antihistamine, without addressing why there was no drainage it may relieve symptoms but not tell you why there is no drainage.
Caleb's parents took him to an ENT specialist which was important and a good thing for them to do considering his snoring. Heavy snoring, tossing, turning and restlessness at night creates an exhausted child during the day.

Tonsils and adenoids help the body to remove viruses and toxins and a tonsillectomy or adenoidectomy are not something to consider doing lightly. Caleb was full of viruses and he was having breathing problems at night. If you are unsure whether this is needed, then get a second opinion. One of my kids had some complications from this surgery because when adding the tubes in the ears the surgeon hit his jugular vein and there was bleeding. After some complications and tests, we still went through with the tonsillectomy and adenoidectomy and he improved just like Caleb. He was alert and willing to learn and picked up more words and phrases. I have interviewed many parents in writing these stories and I have never heard that happen with anyone else. My son's identical twin brother also had mouth breathing but did not snore or get sick like his brother. He did not have surgery and does not need it. My son benefited from this surgery, but always ask questions of your doctors and educate yourself. I chose not to put that in the story because it was not typical, but only as a side note to say that even in identical twins, both don't need the surgery and that this is an individual decision for your family.

Caleb could think clearer, respond and communicate better after being fully rested. He could adapt to the speech, physical and occupational therapy that he needed. A full night's sleep makes an eager learner and checking the child's hearing and eye sight can make a world of difference but it can be overlooked by professionals and teachers and labeled as ADHD.

Advice to Parents with Exhausted Children

Common Reasons for the Children's Exhaustion
If your child is getting adequate rest, there may be medical reasons why they are still exhausted. I've had doctors repeatedly tell me I needed more sleep to the point that I was sleeping too much but I had undiagnosed Lyme disease and that would have saved me years of aggravation. Inflammation in the joints was an indicator for Caleb.
If your child is not getting adequate rest, figure out why. Did they eat, smell, touch or taste anything that might bother them at night?
Your child may not be getting sleep because pain may be keeping him awake. Any type of pain anywhere in his body would keep him awake so a nonverbal child may be holding his stomach would indicate stomach pain which could have several causes.
Read *the Hyper Child* for more help because a child who has not a full night's rest can be overtired and hyper.
Have you ever had an all-nighter studying in college? The exhausted child with Lyme feels like that every day. Real honest autism awareness helps you to understand that feeling and lighten up on the child if he's just too exhausted. He may not just be complaining or lazy but he has a treatable medical condition.
Ear infections and sore throats are not a natural part of childhood. It's so common these days and so many stories of kids like Caleb but that's not normal. It's only become normal since the use of vaccines. Not every kid who has ear infections and sore throats needs a tonsillectomy. A child who isn't breathing properly at night won't sleep and will therefore be exhausted.
Check your child's thyroid if he is wearing a heavy coat when it's hot outside. That may be a key to his exhaustion.

Possible Medical Reasons for the Child's Exhaustion
Candida
Lyme
Parasites
Celiac or gluten intolerance
Some medications used to treat autism
Vaccine injury (a known vaccine injury is fainting)
Mitochondrial dysfunction
Mercury
Aluminum (can cause anemia)
Lead
Allergies
Acute disseminated encephalitis. Brain inflammation that occurs after exposure to a toxin which can happen from a vaccine.

The Depressed or Angry Child
KRISTEN: The Dirt Police

Kristin was a normal 16-year old who liked to clean because it was fun for her. Her homework desk was spotless, her room was spotless and she picked up any loose dirt on the floors with her fingers. She picked up after her little brother and even put things away in her mother's room occasionally. She wouldn't take a shower without it being clean so she cleaned the shower and sink every morning. Her mom bought her plastic gloves to wear while she cleaned because she did not like to touch cleaning products her mother used. She did not like the smells either and asked for a mask like in a hospital to do the cleaning.

Her mother was so proud Kristin was so clean. She never had to ask her to do her homework or to wash dishes because Kristin was happy to do it. She would do extra credit in school for fun and was always looking for more homework when most kids complained. Her hair was always curled the same way and she had it cut every month on the same day like clockwork. Her toenails were always well manicured even though no one ever saw them because she didn't like anything to touch her feet so she never wore open-toed shoes. Kristin washed her hands after every time she cleaned and before she ate, and after using the bathroom and sometimes they just felt dirty and she would just feel that she needed to wash again. Her clothes were perfect and immaculate. Her head had not a hair out of place and of course her hands were clean.

One day Kristin felt a tickle in the back of her throat, and a cough that would not stop. She had a fever and her whole body felt achy and sore. Her throat had white spots in the back of her throat and she was diagnosed with Strep. Kristin's doctor prescribed antibiotics to make her feel better. When she stopped the antibiotics, she still had a sore throat, and her personality had changed. She wasn't happy and joyous anymore. She had become a terrorist house cleaner almost overnight.

She didn't just do a little light housekeeping but now she was ready to use the broom as weapon instead of for sweeping. She wanted to hit anyone with shoes left on the floor or a crooked picture hanging on the wall. After everything that she cleaned, she washed her hands, and continued to do so 10 or 12 times a day. She was a 16-year-old Joan Crawford. She would scream at her family for making a mess and making her clean it up. She screamed at her teachers because their poster on the wall was a little bit crooked. She screamed at her brother for just being in her way. She screamed at everyone who didn't do things exactly as she thought in her mind they should be. "I don't like messes!" she would say to anyone that would listen.

If Kristin had started these outrageous violent behaviors when she was in kindergarten someone might have diagnosed her as ADHD or OCD. Kristin just kept getting suspended and in trouble because she was fighting with everyone. She was bullying other students for being dirty and some kids called her "The Dirt Police" behind her back. Her case is interesting because of the age her symptoms began, a time where such behaviors are often dismissed as typical unruly or angry teenager behavior. In Kristin's case, there was a true medical cause with a solution.

Labels for Kristin

Obsessive Compulsive Behavior is only a problem when it interferes with daily life or takes it over. Medication is not always the answer. Before Kristin had Strep she was successful and orderly but not impulsive or mean. When she reached the threshold of angry and picking fights it was directly after getting a Strep infection. Kristin was labeled as Oppositional Defiant Disorder as well as OCD.

Tools for Kristin and her family

In this case, her anger was the real issue not the obsessive-compulsive disorder. The cleanliness that first described Kristin was not necessarily obsessive-compulsive disorder. You don't have to medicate every single case and it's not all a medical problem. Some people just like things clean. It only becomes a problem when it escalates to anger.

Identify when the anger began. Did she have a real reason to be angry or just explode at everything? It began right after the strep infection. This is a clue for the parents to get a strep test from the doctor to confirm if it's PANDAS. PANDAS means Pediatric Autoimmune Neurologic Disorder Associated with Strep. This is an autoimmune disorder that attacks the part of the brain regulating emotions and kids with PANDAS can be quite angry. PANDAS require a long-term treatment. Some doctors use antibiotics. Some people try homeopathy or a natural method and some use IVIG (Intravenous Immunoglobulin treatments). There are a lot of ways to treat this disorder, but the first step is to get tested.

JENNY: The Fragile Child

Jenny was small for her age and fragile, like a small puppy dog who had been kicked. Everything and everyone seemed to make her cry. Jenny's mother said that Jenny needed Risperdal because she had clinical depression. While she had been just depressed and thought about suicide before taking the drug, now she was planning how to carry it out.

Boys were teasing her because Risperdal made her go through puberty very young and her breasts developed at nine years old. She was more fully developed at ten than most adult females. A short overweight girl with big breasts cannot exactly sit on the sidelines and try to disappear. While she took Risperdal, she became violent and was angry at all the bullying she endured because not only had her breasts grown 4 sizes very quickly but Jenny had gained 40 pounds in just a month.

She had grown like a small infant to a tiny overweight woman in just a month. She would hide under her bed and refuse to go to school for the humiliation she endured for the way she looked. While Jenny looked like a tiny adult female she was still fragile. While some kids fell, and would get a few cuts and scrapes, Jenny would break bones if she fell. Not once, not twice but three times in that year she had gone to the hospital with a broken leg or a broken arm. Jenny was mean to the other kids and refused to play tag or any type of sport because she knew she might get hurt. Teachers thought she was exaggerating and made her play anyway. She was not socializing with other kids. She stayed in her own corner at recess and played by herself. Teachers sent notes home that she was not socializing with other kids at recess and that she often was staring in space during school.

Jenny ate like a bird…always nibbling and never feeling satisfied. She looked at her body and thought she was too heavy. Certain foods made her feel like vomiting especially things with wheat in it, but she didn't know that. She just thought that whatever she ate made her sick and that's because almost all of it contained wheat. When she did eat for a few minutes, she felt better until the food started to digest then she felt sick again. So, she was constantly eating but never very much at a time. She didn't have a full meal of anything, she just nibbled. Even though she ate like she was anorexic, she was a big girl for her age and no one noticed.

Her bones were like they were made from uncooked spaghetti and it seemed like just walking around she was doomed to have a broken bone or two. It happened so often that the nurses at the hospital suspected that Jenny's father was abusive and had called Child Protective Services to take custody of Jenny. Jenny's father was six feet five inches tall a huge man but also with a huge heart. His heart melted around her and loved her dearly and this was not the reason Jenny was so fragile.

Tools For Jenny

Jenny needs to slowly get off the Risperdal. It's dangerous for some of these medications to get off them too quickly and some can make the depression worse. There was a settlement from Johnson and Johnson for $2.2 billion for an off-label use for Risperdal, Invega, and Natrecor. The settlement states that it is an off-label use to market it as an antipsychotic to children. The system makes it difficult for parents to refuse medications however, and it is actually dangerous to stop them too suddenly.

Risperdal has some terrible side effects for children, both males and females because it causes a hormone called lactin which creates gynecomastia which is abnormally large breasts in males, as well as females. The side effects also include pituitary tumors, and involuntary repetitive movements called tardive dyskinesia.

Jenny needed to do a test called a porphyrin test. It will pull the aluminum and other metals out of the organs. This test would prove that her broken bones, bumps and bruises were because of aluminum exposure and not from abuse.

Jenny had full blown celiac and she needed to be gluten free. Some people also feel better going casein free too but for Jenny that did not make much of a difference.

A physical therapist or a customized exercise program that would benefit her. The exercise she needed was slow deep stretches not anything that could get her hurt. Not everyone needs to run and do sports.

Advice to Parents of Depressed or Angry Children

Anger and Depression Labels

These kids might be given all sorts of labels like Depression, Post-Traumatic Stress Disorder, and Anti-Social Personality Disorder. The labels help in getting your child appropriate services and what if any is covered by insurance. I am not suggesting you should label your children differently, or whether any label is considered part of autism or not, but in my experience, effective labels describe the symptoms rather than the core of the situation.

Common Reasons Why a Child on the Spectrum is Angry or Depressed.
Frustration- If your child can't speak or can't speak very clearly, he's frustrated that he isn't heard or getting his point across. He not be able to do things with his body that he knows what to do with his mind.
Fear- Some of the underlying causes create changes in the brain or the fight or flight response to do this even to the mother and father.
Pain-Child who can't communicate his pain may try to tell you in a nonverbal way such as head banging.
Overwhelmed by noise, lack of energy, emotions in the room, bright lights or skin sensitivities. It's as all the senses are overloaded.
Sick-He might even have a fever a sore throat and it's a good idea to check these things when your child isn't cooperating.

Possible Medical Reasons for Anger and Depression
Lyme
Candida
Parasites
Celiac
PANDAS (an autoimmune disease)
Lead
Mercury
Aluminum
Psychiatric drugs
Vitamin deficiency
Allergies
Encephalitis (ADEM)
Artificial colors
Vaccines are linked to autoimmunity, mercury, aluminum, allergies, encephalitis, and vitamin deficiency of which can create a situation where the child is angry. Read Part 4 of this book (on vaccines) for more details.

Part 7: Conclusion

Do Not Comply: Tell the Truth Instead

Doctors say we are better at diagnosing autism, and that's why there is a huge jump in the numbers of kids on the spectrum. I'd say we are better at diagnosing because there are so many more to diagnose. Dr. Stephanie Seneff, PhD (MIT) says in the movie *Vaxxed: From Cover-up to Catastrophe* that if we continue the way we have been, by the year 2032, the rates of autism will be 1 in 2. Half the children and 80% of the boys will be on the spectrum.

As of now, there are no doctors that specialize in autism. There is no program to study autism in any medical college. So, when a doctor from Harvard says he knows all about autism, he did not learn much about it at Harvard because there is no medical specialty in autism and there will not be if medical professionals decide that studying autism will end your medical career. And heaven forbid we find new science to treat it. Autism doctors are behavior specialists like a psychiatrist or psychologist. They are treating the behaviors, and not looking at the medical point of view. There are doctors who specialize in the medial point of view, but they did not go to school to study autism, and instead they found success treating children on the spectrum or even have found treatments for their own kids.

Doctors say they do not study the autism spectrum because there is no cure. There is no cure for cancer either, but there is an entire industry of oncology. Why can't we begin an industry of autism centers and areas for our kids to thrive? We may not be able to cure it, but we could supply a place for them to go and safe place for them to live. They certainly do not need to live with diarrhea, constipation, or in excruciating pain. Yet for many of our kids, these things are fixable.

We are the ones we've been waiting for. The person to teach us about autism is in the mirror. That's me, and that's you. Autism experts are the people who live with it every day, whether they are doctors, parents or both. No one is going to find a placement for our kids, except us. There are not enough group homes, or job opportunities for our kids because we have never had so many grow up at the same time.

I'm asking you to create the life you want for your kid, and tell the world how you did it so that maybe someone else's kid will benefit too. Open autism centers to give adults with autism a place to go. If you own a business, hire a new employee on the spectrum. Train our autism friends in careers, and open more group homes and support other kids who are just like yours.

You have power with your wallet to choose what to buy and where to buy it. You can decide which medications you and your children take, based on the risk versus rewards. You should decide which vaccines to take, which foods to eat and what your family should be exposed to in the environment.

Why are we treating doctors like Gods who can do no wrong? Why are we listening to doctors who are overweight and drinking Diet Coke about nutrition and healthy eating? Health advice from people who are not healthy or don't have healthy habits makes no sense.

You have power to decide who your doctor or dentist will be. There are dentists and doctors that fully understand what is going on with families dealing with toxicity and autism. The dentists that avoid mercury and fluoride are tough to find. There are doctors that will tell you all the benefits and risks of vaccines, and who know and understand Dr. Thompson, and why he is important. You should seek them out.

You also need to take steps to improve your general health. How do you eat better? Grow your own garden, and teach this skill to your children. Schools give tours of the grocery store, not of a farm because the farms are sprayed with Round Up and are too dangerous for children.

Why do we call these poisoned foods conventional and the those that aren't poisoned organic? How about we call them poisoned and not poisoned, or real food and processed food? If there is a natural aisle in your grocery store, what is the rest of the food called? If you want grocery stores to stock better quality foods, don't buy unhealthy foods, no matter how inexpensive they might be. Ask for what you want and look for it. If the stores near you won't supply the food you want, grow it yourself.

Not all of us can jump on a plane and travel city to city and explain to politicians about these things, but that doesn't mean you can't send an email your legislators and explain your story, and ask for services, support and research. And all of us can make a difference in our communities. If all you do is explain to Johnny's teacher why one cookie is not okay for your son, that's one more person in the world who understands something about allergies and toxicity. You've planted a seed.

Some families buy a community of homes in the same neighborhood to share resources, technology and even recipes. Some families buy a farm and share their bounty. Some families stay put but use their computer as the community resource and share via social media.

The educational system, the food system, and career networks all should change as our kids grow up. Every teacher needs to know what is in this book. Our kids need practical training that leads to jobs. Their obsessions can sometimes turn into a career if they have the right teacher.

Kids on the spectrum deserve to be loved, to be independent and to not suffer silently with fatigue, chronic pain, diarrhea or seizures so that they can no longer live with pain. They should not get medication that numbs the pain or sedates them, but should get real treatment, just like anyone else.

The people who do not vaccinate avoid vaccines for a reason and they can go to any school, grocery store they choose and not be prevented from doing so. We are heading down a dangerous road to mandate the same medical care for everyone, because especially with autism, everyone is different.

Now is not the time to cower, or imagine that things will go easier if you just comply. Do we just listen to Nancy Snyderman and "get your damn vaccine?" Or do we step it up, speak out, support our kids, and sharing our story so that it does not happen to everyone else.

Now is the time to make it right. You can do this. We can do this. We are all in this together.

Part 8: APPENDICES

Appendix A: The Stool Chart

Bristol Stool Chart

Type 1	Separate hard lumps like nuts (hard to pass)
Type 2	Sausage-shaped but lumpy
Type 3	Like a sausage but with cracks on the surface
Type 4	Like a sausage or snake, soft and smooth
Type 5	Soft blobs with clear-cut edges
Type 6	Fluffy pieces with ragged edges, a mushy stool
Type 7	Watery, no solid pieces. Entirely liquid

http://static1.1.sqspcdn.com/static/f/1451532/22180508/1363249562587/bristol_stool_chart.pdf

Appendix B: Yeast Symptoms

Headaches	Laughing at the wrong time	Sleeping Issues
Crying issues	Stomach ache	Constipation
Bed wetting	Gas pains	Fatigue
Depression	Brain fog	Attention deficit
Hyperactivity	Anger	Stimming
Squealing	Sensory issues	Climbing
Sugar Cravings	Confusion	Lethargy
Not potty trained	Craving certain foods	Missed developmental milestones
Rashes on the skin	Rash on the mouth	Red ring on the anus
Rash between the toes		

http://www.tacanow.org/family-resources/what-is-yeast-overgrowth/
A comprehensive list of remedies to treat yeast is available here.

Appendix C: Always Eat Organic

Apple	Strawberry
Nectarine	Peach
Celery	Grapes
Cherries	Spinach
Tomatoes	Sweet Bell Peppers
Cherry Tomatoes	Cucumbers

Environmental Working Group Dirty Dozen

Appendix D: Ingredients That Contain MSG

Glutamic Acid E620	Monosodium Glutamate E621
Calcium Glutamate E623	Monoammonium Glutamate E 624
Magnesium Glutamate E 624	Natrium Glutamate
Anything hydrolyzed	Any Hydrolyzed protein
Calcium Caseinate or Sodium Caseinate	Yeast Extract or Torula Yeast
Yeast Food or Yeast Nutrient	Autolyzed yeast
Gelatin	Whey Protein
Whey Protein Concentrate	Whey Protein Isolate
Soy Protein	Soy Protein Concentrate
Soy Protein isolate	Anything Protein
Anything Protein fortified	Soy Sauce
Soy Sauce Extract	Anything enzyme modified
Anything containing enzymes	Anything fermented
Anything containing protease	Vetsin
Anjinomoto	Umami

Appendix E: Ingredients That May Contain MSG

Carrageenan (E 407)	Oligodextrin
Bouillon and broth	Citric Acid
Stock	Anything Ultra Pasteurized
Any "flavors" or "flavoring"	Barley Malt
Natural flavor	Malted Barley
Maltodextrin	Brewer's Yeast
Seasonings	

http://www.truthinlabeling.org/hiddensources.html

Appendix F: Comparison Chart for Symptoms of MS, Lyme Disease, Fibromyalgia and CFS

Multiple Sclerosis	Lyme Disease
Awkward gait	Anxiety
Bladder dysfunction	Bowel dysfunction
Bowel dysfunction	Breathing issues (air hunger)
Breathing issues	Cardiac issues
Cognitive dysfunction	Confusion
Depression	Depression
Dizziness	Difficulty finding words
Emotional changes	Disorientation/getting lost
Fatigue	Disturbed sleep
Headache	Dizziness/light-headedness
Hearing loss	Ears ringing or buzzing
Itching	Enlarged lymph nodes
Numbness	Facial paralysis (Bell's Palsy)
Pain	Fatigue
Seizures	Fever/sweats/chills
Sexual dysfunction	Forgetfulness
Spasticity	Headache
Speech disorders	Intolerance to alcohol
Swallowing problems	Irritability/mood changes
Tremors	Irritable bladder
Vertigo	Joint pain & swelling
Vision problems	Migrating pain
	Neck pain & cracking
SOURCE: nationalMSsociety.org	Muscular pain
	Pelvic pain
	Numbness & tingling
	Sexual dysfunction
	Skin sensitivity
	Sound/light/smell intolerance
	Seizures
	Breast or testicular pain
	Tremor/twitching
	Unavoidable need to lie down
	Vision issues/blurry/double vision
	SOURCE: Diagnostic Hints & Treatment Guidelines for Lyme & Other Tick-borne illnesses, Joseph J. Burrascano, MD

Fibromyalgia	Chronic Fatigue Syndrome
Anxiety	Enlarged lymph nodes
Depression	Inability to exercise
Breathing issues (sleep apnea)	Exhaustion
Fatigue	Fatigue
Pain/pressure points	Headache
- Back of head	Memory loss
- Between shoulder blades	Poor concentration
- Top of shoulders	Migrating pain
- Front side of neck	Muscle pain
- Upper chest	Sleeping disturbance
- Outer elbows	Sore throat
- Upper hips	
- Side of hips	
- Inner knees	
Restless legs	
Sleep disturbances	

SOURCE: http://www.mayoclinic.org/diseases-conditions/fibromyalgia/basics/symptoms/con-20019243

SOURCE: www.mayoclinic.org/diseases-conditions/chronic-fatigue-syndrome/basics/definition/con-20022009

Symptom Comparison Chart

Appendix G: Common Signs of Toxicity from Dr. Doris Rapp

Physical	Behavioral	Educational
Wrinkles below the eyes	Fatigue	Sloppy handwriting
Swollen cracked lips	Refusal to follow directions	Lower IQ scores
Nausea, bloating, constipation	Can't sit still	Changes in speech
Wiggling legs or arms	Easily distracted	Change in coordination

(The Impossible Child by Doris Rapp MD, FAAA, FAAP Practical Life Allergy Research Foundation 1986)

Appendix H: 15 Toxic Occupations

Refuse and Recyclable Material Collectors	Nuclear Operation Technician
Medical, Clinical and Cardiovascular Technologist or Technician	Pilot, Copilot and Flight Engineers
Oil and Gas Operators	Surgical Technicians
Stationary Engineers and Boiler Operators	Waste and Waste Water System Operators
Immigration and Custom Inspectors	Podiatrists
Veterinary and Veterinary Assistants	Anesthesiologist, Nurse Anesthesiologist or Anesthesiologist Assistants
Flight Attendant	Dentist, Dental Hygienists and Dental Lab Technicians
Histotechnologist and Histotechnologists Assistance	

Business Insider The 15 jobs that are the most damaging to your health

Appendix I: US Mortality Rates for Polio, Smallpox, Diptheria, & Typhoid

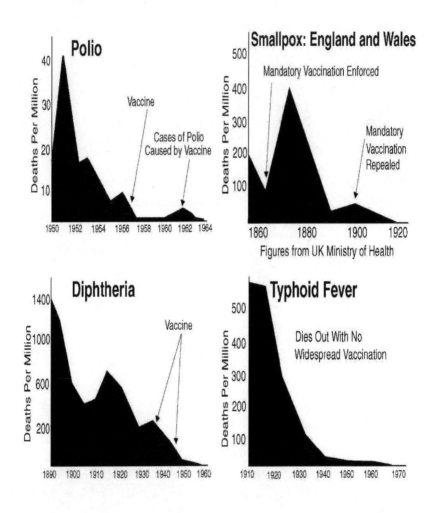

Appendix J: Vaccine Information Statement vs. Vaccine Insert

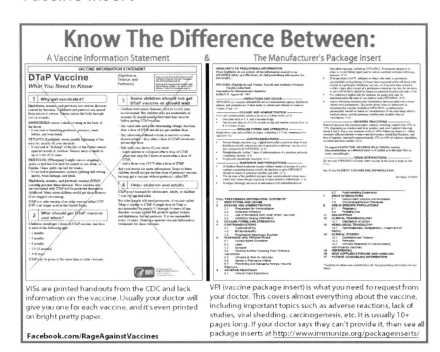

http://www.immunize.org/packageinserts/

Appendix K: 28 studies from around the world that support Dr. Wakefield's controversial findings:

1. The Journal of Pediatrics November 1999; 135(5):559-63
2. The Journal of Pediatrics 2000; 138(3): 366-372
3. Journal of Clinical Immunology November 2003; 23(6): 504-517
4. Journal of Neuroimmunology 2005
5. Brain, Behavior and Immunity 1993; 7: 97-103
6. Pediatric Neurology 2003; 28(4): 1-3
7. Neuropsychobiology 2005; 51:77-85
8. The Journal of Pediatrics May 2005;146(5):605-10
9. Autism Insights 2009; 1: 1-11
10. Canadian Journal of Gastroenterology February 2009; 23(2): 95-98
11. Annals of Clinical Psychiatry 2009:21(3): 148-161
12. Journal of Child Neurology June 29, 2009; 000:1-6
13. Journal of Autism and Developmental Disorders March 2009;39(3):405-1
14. Medical Hypotheses August 1998; 51:133-144.
15. Journal of Child Neurology July 2000; ;15(7):429-35
16. Lancet. 1972; 2:883–884.
17. Journal of Autism and Childhood Schizophrenia January-March 1971; 1:48-62
18. Journal of Pediatrics March 2001;138:366-372.
19. Molecular Psychiatry 2002;7:375-382.
20. American Journal of Gastroenterology April 2004;598-605.
21. Journal of Clinical Immunology November 2003;23:504-517.
22. Neuroimmunology April 2006;173(1-2):126-34.
23. Prog. Neuropsychopharmacol Biol. Psychiatry December

30 2006;30:1472-1477.
24. Clinical Infectious Diseases September 1 2002;35(Suppl 1):S6-S16
25. Applied and Environmental Microbiology, 2004;70(11):6459-6465
26. Journal of Medical Microbiology October 2005;54:987-991
27. Archivos venezolanos de puericultura y pediatría 2006; Vol 69 (1): 19-25
28. Gastroenterology. 2005:128 (Suppl 2); Abstract-303

Appendix L: Behavior Chart

Date	Breakfast	Lunch	Dinner	What Happened?	Duration	Possible cause?

Appendix M: State Vaccine Exemptions

State	Medical	Religious	Philosophical
Alabama	X	X	
Alaska	X	X	
Arizona	X	X	X
Arkansas	X	X	X
California	X		
Colorado	X	X	X
Connecticut	X	X	
Delaware	X	X	
Florida	X	X	
Georgia	X	X	
Hawaii	X	X	
Idaho	X	X	X
Illinois	X	X	
Indiana	X	X	
Iowa	X	X	
Kansas	X	X	
Kentucky	X	X	
Louisiana	X	X	X
Maine	X	X	X
Massachusetts	X	X	
Michigan	X	X	X
Minnesota	X	X	X
Mississippi	X		
Missouri	X	X	
Montana	X	X	

State	Medical	Religious	Philosophical
Nebraska	X	X	
Nevada	X	X	
New Hampshire	X	X	
New Jersey	X	X	
New Mexico	X	X	
New York	X	X	
North Carolina	X	X	
North Dakota	X	X	X
Ohio	X	X	X
Oklahoma	X	X	X
Oregon	X	X	X
Pennsylvania	X	X	
Rhode Island	X	X	
South Carolina	X	X	
South Dakota	X	X	
Tennessee	X	X	
Texas	X	X	X
Utah	X	X	X
Vermont	X	X	
Virginia	X	X	
Washington	X	X	X
West Virginia	X		
Wisconsin	X	X	X
Wyoming	X	X	

Appendix N: Vaccines that Contain Aborted Fetal Cells (reasons for religious exemptions)

Michigan Right to Life

Disease	Vaccine Name	Manufacturer	Cell line
Adenovirus		Barr Labs., Inc.	WI-38
Chickenpox	Varivax	Merck & Co.	MRC-5 & WI-38
Diphtheria, Tetanus, Pertussis, Polio, HIB	Pentacel	Sanofi Pasteur	MRC-5
Hepatitis A	Havrix	GlaxoSmithKline	MRC-5
Hepatitis A	Vaqta	Merck & Co.	MRC-5
Hepatitis A-B	Twinrix	GlaxoSmithKline	MRC-5
Measles, Mumps, Rubella	MMR II	Merck & Co.	WI-38
Measles, Mumps, Rubella, Chickenpox	ProQuad	Merck & Co.	MRC-5 & WI-38
Rabies	Imovax	Sanofi Pasteur	MRC-5
Shingles	Zostavax	Merck & Co.	MRC-5

Appendix O: Recommended Books

Books about the Gut

Bugs Bowels and Behavior, The Groundbreaking Story of the Gut Brain Connection by Teri Arranga, Claire Viadro, Lauren Underwood and Martha Herbert. Skyhorse Publishing 2013

What's Eating Your Child, The Hidden Connections between Food and Childhood Ailments: Anxiety, Recurrent Ear Infections, Stomachaches, Picky Eating, Rashes, ADHD and More. What Every Parent Can do About it. By Kelly Dorfman Workman Publishing 2011

Toxicity Books

Poisoned Profits, The Toxic Assault on our Children by Phillip an Alice Shabecoff Random House 2008

The Impossible Child, A Guide for Caring Teachers and Parents in School and at Home by Doris Rapp MD FAA FAAP

Vaccines

Vaccine Whistleblower, Exposing The Research Fraud at the CDC by Kevin Barry Skyhorse publishing 2015

Vaccine Epidemic, How Corporate Greed, Biased Science and Coercive Government Threatens Our Human Rights, Our Health and Our Children by Louise Habakus MA and Mary Holland JD Skyhorse Publishing 2011

Recommended Movies

Vaxxed: From Cover-up to Catastrophe

Trace Amounts

Diet Books

Candida

The Complete Candida Yeast Guidebook, Everything You Need to Know About Prevention Treatment and Diet by Zoltan Rona MD

MSG

The Slow Poisoning of America by John Erb Paladins Press 2003

Paleo

Everyday Paleo by Sarah Fragoso Victory Press Publishing 2011

GFCF

Celeste Best Gluten free, allergen free recipes, over 250 recipes free of Gluten, wheat, dairy casein soy by Celeste Clevenger Luminary Publications 2012

End Notes

Part 1: The Gut, The Brain and the Immune System

[1] Miralax FDA Potential Signals of Serious Risk/New Safety Information Identified by the Adverse Event Reporting System AERS Between October and December 2011. https://www.fda.gov/Drugs/GuidanceComplianceRegulatoryInformation/Surveillance/AdverseDrugEffects/ucm295585.htm

[2] Macintosh, James. *Serotonin Facts: What does Serotonin do?* Medical News Today. http://www.medicalnewstoday.com/kc/serotonin-facts-232248

[3] Prandovszky, E., et.al. *Neuropsychiatric disease and Toxoplasma Gondii Infection.* PLOS. 2009 Feb 11. http://journals.plos.org/plosone/article?id=10.1371/journal.pone.0023866

[4] Muille, Jennifer. *The Gut Microbe: A New Frontier in Autism Research.* Current Psychiatry Rep. Feb 1 2014. https://www.ncbi.nlm.nih.gov/pmc/articles/PMC3564498/

[5] McMillen, Matt. *Leaky Gut Syndrome: What is it? What you should know if you have Leaky Gut Syndrome.* WebMD. http://www.webmd.com/digestive-disorders/features/leaky-gut-syndrome#1

[6] Gershon, Michael. *The Second Brain: The Scientific Basis of Gut Instinct and Groundbreaking New Understanding of Nervous Disorders of the Stomach and Intestines.* NY: Harper Perennial, 1999

[7] Ibid.

[8] Barney, Josh. *They'll Have to Rewrite the Textbooks.* March 21, 2016
https://news.virginia.edu/illimitable/discovery/theyll-have-rewrite-textbooks

[9] Coury, Daniel. Gastrointestinal Conditions in Children with Autism Spectrum Disorder Developing a Research Agenda. American Academy of Pediatrics. 130(2) Nov 2012.

[10] Nikolov, Roumen. Gastrointestinal Symptoms in a Sample of Children with Pervasive Developmental Disorders. J Autism Dev Disord. 2008

[11] Hausteiner-Wiehle, Constanze. *Irritable Bowel Syndrome: Relations with functional, mental and somataform disorders.* World Journal of Gastroenterology. May 28, 2014.

[12] Gut and Psychology Syndrome Dr Natasha McBride GAPS Syndrome or GAPS

[13] Arranga, Terri. Bugs, Bowels and Behavior: The Groundbreaking Story of the Gut Brain Connection. NY: Skyhorse Publishing, 2013

[14] Horvath, K., et. al. *Gastrointestinal Abnormalities in Children with Autistic Disorder.* Journal of Pediatrics. 1999 Nov;135(5):559-63.
https://www.ncbi.nlm.nih.gov/pubmed/10547242

[15] Arranga, Terri. Bugs, Bowels and Behavior: The Groundbreaking Story of the Gut Brain Connection. NY: Skyhorse Publishing, 2013

[16] *Potty Training Readiness Checklist.* Baby Center Blog. July, 2016. http://www.babycenter.com/0_potty-training-readiness-checklist_4384.bc

[17] Singh S Low Plazma Zinc and Iron in PICA
https://www.ncbi.nlm.nih.gov/pubmed/12661808

[18] Kumamoto, Carol. *Inflammation and Gastrointestinal Candida Colonization*. Current Opinions in Microbiology. 2011; Aug;14(4):386-91.
https://www.ncbi.nlm.nih.gov/pubmed/21802979

[19] Bortfeld, Holly. *What is Yeast Overgrowth?* Talk about Curing Autism. November 23, 2015.
http://www.tacanow.org/family-resources/what-is-yeast-overgrowth/

[20] Ibid.

[21] Great Plains Laboratory Comprehensive Stool Analysis
https://www.greatplainslaboratory.com/comprehensive-stool-analysis/

[22] CDC Invasive Candidasis
https://www.nlm.nih.gov/medlineplus/ency/article/000818.htm

[23] Boyle, RJ The Clinical Syndrome of Specific antibody deficiency of children 3 Nov 2006
http://onlinelibrary.wiley.com/doi/10.1111/j.1365-2249.2006.03242.x/full

[24] Round Up and GMOs: Are we Gambling with the Future of Foods Stephanie Seneff MIT CSAIL July 29, 2014
https://people.csail.mit.edu/seneff/glyphosate/Taiwan_July2014.pdf

[25] Hornlein, Carol. MSGTruth.org

[26] Swaminathan Nikhi Largest Gene Identified: Two Genetic Culprits Feb 18, 2007 Nature America
https://www.scientificamerican.com/article/largest-autism-study-finds-two-genes/

[27] Questions and Answers on Monosodium Glutamate (MSG) November 19, 2012 FDA
https://www.fda.gov/Food/IngredientsPackagingLabeling/FoodAdditivesIngredients/ucm328728.htm

[28] Hornlein, Carol. MSGTruth.org

[29] Zoltan, Rona. *Altered Immunity and Leaky Gut Syndrome.* Foods Matter. nd.
http://www.foodsmatter.com/digestive_conditions/miscellaneous/articles/leaky-gut-rona-eir-08-12.html

[30] Schoenthaler, S.J. *The Effect of Vitamin Supplementation on Juvenile Delinquency among American School Children; A Randomized Double Blind Placebo Controlled Trial* Journal of Alternative Complementary Medicine. 2000 Feb;6(1):7-17.
https://www.ncbi.nlm.nih.gov/pubmed/10706231

[31] Gesch, C. B., et. al. *Influence of Supplementary Vitamins, Minerals, and Essential Fatty Acids on the Antisocial Behavior of Young Adult Prisoners; A Random Placebo Controlled Trial.* Journal of Psychiatry. 2002 Jul;181:22-8
.https://www.ncbi.nlm.nih.gov/pubmed/12091259

[32] Medline Plus. *Pica.* nd.
https://www.nlm.nih.gov/medlineplus/ency/article/001538.htm

[33] WebMD. *Vitamin D Deficiency.* nd.
http://www.webmd.com/diet/guide/vitamin-d-deficiency

[34] Gabaeff, Steven *Challenging the Pathophysiological Connection between Subdural Hematona, Retinal Hemorrhage and Shake Baby Syndrome* 2011 May
https://www.ncbi.nlm.nih.gov/pmc/articles/PMC3099599/

[35] Clemetson, C. Alan B. *Shaken Baby Syndrome or Scurvy.* Journal of Orthomolecular Medicine. Vol. 17, No. 4, 2002; 193-196.
http://www.orthomolecular.org/library/jom/2002/pdf/2002-v17n04-p193.pdf

[36] Seneff, Stephanie. *Is Encephalopathy a Mechanism to Renew Sulfate in Autism.* Entropy 2013, 15, 372-406.
https://people.csail.mit.edu/seneff/Entropy/entropy-15-00372.pdf

Part 2: How Does Lyme Disease Affect Behavior and Physical Health?

[37] Ticks and Lyme Disease, Pregnancy and Lyme Disease CDC
https://www.cdc.gov/lyme/resources/toolkit/factsheets/10_508_lyme-disease_pregnantwoman_factsheet.pdf

[38] Eckholm, Eric. *Caution is Urged on Lyme Vaccine for Dogs.* New York Times. June 22, 1991.
http://www.nytimes.com/1991/06/22/news/caution-is-urged-on-lyme-disease-vaccinations-for-dogs.html

[39] Bransfield, R.C. *The Association Between Tick Born Infections, Lyme Borreliosis and Autism Spectrum Disorders.* Med Hypothesis. 2008;70(5):967-74
https://www.ncbi.nlm.nih.gov/pubmed/17980971

[40] Centers for Disease Control. *CDC Provides Estimate of Americans Diagnosed with Lyme Disease Each Year.* Press Release. August 19, 2013.
http://www.cdc.gov/media/releases/2013/p0819-lyme-disease.html

[41] Kugeler, J. *A Review of Death Certificates Listing Lyme Disease as a Cause of Death in the United States.* Clin Infect Dis. *(2011) 52 (3): 364-367.*
http://cid.oxfordjournals.org/content/52/3/364.full

[42] CDC. *Lyme Disease.* nd. http://www.cdc.gov/lyme/

[43] Todar, K. *Borrelia burgdorferi and Lyme Disease.* nd. Online Textbook of Bacteriology.
http://textbookofbacteriology.net/Lyme.html

[44] Melaun, C., et. al. *Occurrence of Borrelia Burdoferi s.l. in Different Genera of Mosquitoes (Culicidae) in Central Europe.* Ticks and Tick-borne Diseases. 7(2). March 2016, Pages 256–263.
http://www.sciencedirect.com/science/journal/1877959X/7/2

[45] Lyme Disease Can be Sexually Transmitted: Study Suggests PR web
Carmel CA January 25, 2014
http://www.prweb.com/releases/2014/01/prweb11506441.htm

[46] CDC Lyme Disease Frequently Asked Questions.
https://www.cdc.gov/lyme/faq/

[47] Bransfield, R.C. *The Association Between Tick Born Infections, Lyme Borreliosis and Autism Spectrum Disorders.* Med Hypothesis. 2008;70(5):967-74.
https://www.ncbi.nlm.nih.gov/pubmed/17980971

[48] CDC. *Lyme: Signs and Symptoms.* nd.
http://www.cdc.gov/lyme/signs_symptoms/index.html

[49] Columbia University Medical Center: Lyme and Tick-Borne Diseases Research Center. *Symptoms and Signs.* nd. http://columbia-lyme.org/patients/ld_lyme_symptoms.html

[50] *An Understanding of Laboratory Testing for Lyme Disease.* Journal of Spirochetal and Tick-borne Diseases. Vol. 5, Spring/Summer 1998. http://www.igenex.com/labtest.htm

[51] Grier, Tom. *Will There Ever Be an Accurate Test for Lyme Disease?* Self-Published Reference Booklet. http://www.lymemed.nl/discussie/grier.pdf

[52] CDC. *Notice to Readers Recommendations for Test Performance and Interpretation from the Second National Conference on Serologic Diagnosis of Lyme Disease* Aug 11, 1995. http://www.cdc.gov/mmwr/preview/mmwrhtml/00038469.htm

[53] Occupy US DOJ. *Lymerix, Vaccines and Immunosuppression.* Video. https://vimeo.com/channels/cryme/180648200

[54] Sheller, Ludwig & Badey. Submission for January 31, 2001 Advisory Committee Meeting. Private letter. January 24, 2001. http://www.fda.gov/ohrms/dockets/ac/01/briefing/3680b2_21.pdf

[55] Nigrovic, L.E. *The Lyme Vaccine: A Cautionary Tale.* Epidemiology and Infection. 2007 Jan; 135(1): 1–8. https://www.ncbi.nlm.nih.gov/pmc/articles/PMC2870557/

[56] Berghoff, Walter. *Chronic Lyme Disease Co Infections: Differential Diagnosis.* Open Neurology. 2012;6:158-78. https://www.ncbi.nlm.nih.gov/pubmed/23400696

[57] *Babesia.* LymeDisease. org. nd.
https://www.lymedisease.org/lyme-basics/co-infections/babesia/

[58] *Bartonella.* LymeDisease.org. nd.
https://www.lymedisease.org/lyme-basics/co-infections/bartonella/

[59] University of Leeds. *Brain Parasite Directly Effects Brain Chemistry.* Science Daily. Nov 7, 2011.
https://www.sciencedaily.com/releases/2011/11/111104102125.htm

[60] Abdoli A. *Are there any relationships between latent Toxoplasma Gondii Infection, Testosterone and Autism Spectrum Disorder?* Frontiers in Behavioral Neuroscience. 2014; 8: 339.
https://www.ncbi.nlm.nih.gov/pmc/articles/PMC4173877/

[61] Snyder, Bill. *Altered Dopamine Signaling May Offer a Clue in Autism.* Research News at Vanderbilt. Jan 29, 2015.
https://news.vanderbilt.edu/2015/01/29/altered-dopamine-signaling-may-offer-a-clue-to-autism/.

[62] CDC. *Mycoplasma pneumoniae Infection.* nd.
http://www.cdc.gov/pneumonia/atypical/mycoplasma/

[63] CDC. *Tickborne Diseases of the United States.* nd.
http://www.cdc.gov/ticks/diseases/.

[64] CDC. *Post-Treatment Lyme Disease Syndrome.* nd.
https://www.cdc.gov/lyme/postlds/

[65] ILADS. *Ilads Physician Referral Form.*
http://ilads.org/ilads_media/physician-referral/.

Part 3: Toxicity: How does Environment Affect Behavior

[66] Urine Porphyrins. Doctor's Data: Science and Insight.. nd https://www.doctorsdata.com/urine-porphyrins/.

[67] Shabecoff, A. and P. *Poisoned Profits: The Toxic Assault on our Children.* NY: Random House, 2008.

[68] Rettner, R. *Epigenetics: Definition and Examples.* Live Science. June 24, 2013. http://www.livescience.com/37703-epigenetics.html.

[69] Robertson, Sally. What is DNA Methylation? News Medical & Life Sciences. December 7,2016 .http://www.news-medical.net/life-sciences/What-is-DNA-Methylation.aspx

[70] Ibid.

[71] Boris, Marvin, et.al. *Associations of MTHFR Gene Variants with Autism.* Journal of American Physicians and Surgeons. 9(4); Winter 2004. 106-108. http://www.jpands.org/vol9no4/boris.pdf

[72] Ibid.

[73] Ibid.

[74] Kelly, R., & Krieger, K. *Subject: Abnormalities in Mitochondrial Metabolism in Children with Pervasive Developmental Disorder* Johns Hopkins and Cleveland Clinic.

[75] Sircus, Doctor. *Mitochondrial Medicine.* May 23, 2013. http://drsircus.com/medicine/mitochondrial-medicine-cocktails/

[76] Meyer, J., et. al. *Mitochondria as Targets of Environmental Toxicants* Toxicological Sciences. *Toxicol. Sciences.* April 29, 2013. http://toxsci.oxfordjournals.org/content/early/2013/05/22/toxsci.kft102.full.html

[77] Ibid.

[78] James, S.L. *Thimerosal Neurotoxicity is Associated with Glutathione Depletion: Protection with Glutathione Precursors* Neurotoxicology. 29(1) 2005. 108.

[79] Mercury Exposure. *Boyd Haley Ph.D. explains the link between APOE4 and genetic susceptibility to mercury toxicity.* Video. https://youtu.be/922vQfyHe7o

[80] Seipjere. *Dr. Boyd Haley: Autism, Mercury & Thimerosal.* 2005. Video. https://youtu.be/anirpRdz8I8

[81] Mikovits, J. *Environmental Causes of Autism. Investigate if You Dare.* Autism One. July 28, 2014. http://www.autismone.org/content/environmental-causes-autism-investigate-if-you-dare-dr-judy-mikovits

[82] *Tuberous Sclerosis Fact Sheet.* National Institute of Neurological Disorders and Stroke. nd. http://www.ninds.nih.gov/disorders/tuberous_sclerosis/detail_tuberous_sclerosis.htm

[83] Atkinson, S. *Learning from a Previous Vaccine-Autism Case.* CBS News. Aug 1 2008. http://www.cbsnews.com/news/learning-from-a-previous-vaccine-autism-case/

[84] Environmental Working Group. *Body Burden: The Pollution of Newborns.* July 14, 2005. http://www.ewg.org/research/body-burden-pollution-newborns

[85] CDC. *Reproductive Health: Preterm Birth.* nd. http://www.cdc.gov/reproductivehealth/maternalinfanthealth/pretermbirth.htm

[86] Cell Press. *Study uncovers why autism is more common in males.* Science Daily. Feb 27, 2014. https://www.sciencedaily.com/releases/2014/02/140227125236.htm

[87] *Autism Spectrum Disorder (ASD).* National Institute of Mental Health. https://www.nimh.nih.gov/health/statistics/prevalence/autism-spectrum-disorder-asd.shtml

[88] IAOMT. *Smoking Teeth=Toxic Fillings.* Jan 23, 2011. https://youtu.be/Bw94F94FZqA

[89] Haley, B. *Letter to the Honorable Dan Burton Responding to ADA President.* Personal Correspondence. 23 May 2001. http://www.fda.gov/ohrms/dockets/dailys/02/Sep02/091602/80027dd6.pdf

[90] *Statement on Dental Amalgam.* nd. American Dental Association. http://www.ada.org/en/about-the-ada/ada-positions-policies-and-statements/statement-on-dental-amalgam.

[91] *Dental Effluent Guidelines.* EPA. October 21, 2016. https://www.epa.gov/eg/dental-effluent-guidelines.

[92] *Disposal of Waste: Outdated Vaccine.* Colorado Department of Public Health and Environment. December, 2010. https://www.colorado.gov/pacific/sites/default/files/HM_mw-waste-outdated-vaccine.pdf.

[93] Center for Environmental Health

[94] *Protect Your Family from Lead in the Home.* nd. EPA Lead Protect your Family. https://www.epa.gov/lead/protect-your-family-lead-your-home

[95] Harding, Anne. *Antidepressant Use in Pregnancy May Raise Autism Risk.* CNN. July 6, 201. http://www.cnn.com/2011/HEALTH/07/04/antidepressant.pregnancy.autism.risk/

[96] Perna R. Terbutaline and Associated Risk for Neurodevelopmental disorders Child Development Research Vol 22014 Article ID 358608 https://www.hindawi.com/journals/cdr/2014/358608/

[97] Shaw, William. *Increased Acetaminophen use appears to be a major cause of the epidemics of autism, ADHD and Asthma.* Great Plains Laboratory. Oct 30, 2013. https://www.greatplainslaboratory.com/articles-1/2015/11/13/evidence-that-increased-acetaminophen-use-in-genetically-vulnerable-children-appears-to-be-a-major-cause-of-the-epidemics-of-autism-attention-deficit-with-hyperactivity-and-asthma.

[98] Schultz, S.T,. et. al. *Acetaminophen (Paracetamol) Use, Measles, Mumps Rubella Vaccination, and Autistic Disorder: The Results of a Parent Survey.* Autism. 2008 May;12(3):293-307. https://www.ncbi.nlm.nih.gov/pubmed/18445737

[99] *Lead Levels Linked to Lower IQ Levels in Children.* ABC News. June 2, ny. http://abcnews.go.com/GMA/AmericanFamily/story?id=125121&page=1

[100] A Different Kind of School Lunch Applegate Wisconsin http://www.feingold.org/PF/wisconsin1.html

[101] Nutritional Influences on Aggressive Behaviors Werbach, Melvyn R Orthomelecular.org Journal of Orthomolecular Medicine 1995
http://www.orthomolecular.org/library/articles/webach.shtml

[102] Ayatollahi, J., et. al. *Occupational Hazards to Dental Staff.* Dental Research Journal. 2012 Jan-Mar; 9(1): 2–7.
https://www.ncbi.nlm.nih.gov/pmc/articles/PMC3283973/

[103] CDC. *Artificial Turf.* nd.
https://www.cdc.gov/nceh/lead/tips/artificialturf.htm

[104] Genova Diagnostics Porphyrins-Urine
https://www.gdx.net/product/porphyrins-test-urine

[105] Miller, A.L. Dimercaptosuccinic acid (DMSA), a non-toxic, water-soluble treatment for heavy metal toxicity. Alternative Medicine Rev. 1998 Jun;3(3):199-207.
https://www.ncbi.nlm.nih.gov/pubmed/9630737

[106] Organic Acids Test (OAT) Nutritional & Metabolic Profile. The Great Plains Laboratory. nd.
http://www.greatplainslaboratory.com/organic-acids-test

Part 4: Why are Vaccines So Controversial?

[107] MYC-Span Clip. Testing Autism between Vaccinated and Unvaccinated Children. Cable Website. November 29, 2012.
http://www.c-span.org/video/?c4201064/testing-autism-vaccinated-unvaccinated-children

[108] Posey Questions CDC on Vaccine Research Congressman Posey November 29, 2012
https://youtu.be/uNWTOmEi_6A

[109] Highlights of Prescribing Information: Flumist. FDA. nd.
http://www.fda.gov/downloads/BiologicsBloodVaccines/Vaccines/ApprovedProducts/UCM294307.pdf

[110] Medical Errors are #3 Cause of US Death: Researchers Say NPR May 3, 2016
http://www.npr.org/sections/health-shots/2016/05/03/476636183/death-certificates-undercount-toll-of-medical-errors

[111] *Highlights of Prescribing Information: Flulaval.* FDA. nd.
http://www.fda.gov/downloads/BiologicsBloodVaccines/Vaccines/ApprovedProducts/UCM112904.pdf

[112] Highlights of Prescribing Information: Flumist. FDA. nd.
http://www.fda.gov/downloads/BiologicsBloodVaccines/Vaccines/ApprovedProducts/UCM294307.pdf

[113] Vaccine Information Statement for HPV
https://www.cdc.gov/vaccines/hcp/vis/vis-statements/hpv.pdf

[114] http://www.merriam-webster.com/dictionary/immune

[115] Palmer, Kim. *Ohio Mumps Outbreak Grows To 116 Cases, Mainly At Ohio State University.* Huffington Post. April 1, 2014. http://www.huffingtonpost.com/2014/04/02/ohio-mumps-outbreak-ohio-state-university_n_5072257.html

[116] Gergana, Koleva. *Merck Whistleblower Suit A Boon to Vaccine Foes Even as it Stresses Importance of Vaccines.* Forbes Magazine. June 27, 2012.
http://www.forbes.com/sites/gerganakoleva/2012/06/27/merck-whistleblower-suit-a-boon-to-anti-vaccination-advocates-though-it-stresses-importance-of-vaccines/

[117] Osterholm, M.T. *Infectious Diseases, Efficacy and Effectiveness of Influenza Vaccines, A Systemic Review and Meta-Analysis.* The Lancet. Oct 26, 2011. p. 36–44.
http://www.thelancet.com/journals/laninf/article/PIIS1473-3099(11)70295-X/abstract

[118] *Highlights of Prescribing Information: Flulaval.* FDA. nd. http://www.fda.gov/downloads/BiologicsBloodVaccines/Vaccines/ApprovedProducts/UCM112904.pdf

[119] Recommended Immunization Schedule for Children and Adolescents age 18 Years and Younger CDC 2017 https://www.cdc.gov/vaccines/schedules/hcp/imz/child-adolescent-compliant.html

[120] Manookian, Leslie, et. al. Frequently Asked Questions: The Greater Good Movie.

[121] Recommended Immunization Schedule for Children and Adolescents age 18 Years and Younger CDC 2017 https://www.cdc.gov/vaccines/schedules/hcp/imz/child-adolescent-compliant.html

[122] Acosta, A.M., et. al. *Long Term Efficacy Rates for Pertussis following TDAP, Recent Whooping Cough Epidemics among Adolescents.* Cleveland Clinic Journal of Medicine. June 30, 2015. http://www.ccjm.org/clinicaledge/vaccines-public-health/single-article/long-term-efficacy-rates-for-pertussis-following-tdap/a472a117beae537686fe00eec3c32429.html

[123] Blaylock, Russell. *Forced Vaccinations, Government and the Public Interest part 1. Is Herd Immunity Real?* The Epoch Times. December 27, 2009. http://www.theepochtimes.com/n2/health/forced-vaccinations-government-and-the-public-interest-2-27045.html

[124] Senate Bill SB277 California https://leginfo.legislature.ca.gov/faces/billNavClient.xhtml?bill_id=201520160SB277

[125] *Senate Bill No. 792: Chapter 807.* California Legislative Information. October 11, 2015. https://leginfo.legislature.ca.gov/faces/billNavClient.xhtml?bill_id=201520160SB792

[126] Wilson, Federica S. *H.R.2232 — 114th Congress (2015-2016).* https://www.congress.gov/bill/114th-congress/house-bill/2232/text

[127] Offit, Paul, et. al. *Addressing Parents' Concerns: Do Multiple Vaccines Overwhelm or Weaken the Infant's Immune System?* American Academy of Pediatrics. January 1, 2002. http://pediatrics.aappublications.org/content/109/1/124.full

[128] Frontline. "The Vaccine War." April 27, 2010. http://www.pbs.org/wgbh/pages/frontline/vaccines/interviews/offit.html

[129] Minnesota Department of Health. *Ensuring Immunity to Varicella in Health Care Workers.* nd. http://www.health.state.mn.us/divs/idepc/diseases/varicella/hcp/hcwimmunity.html.

[130] *Piers Morgan Gets a Flu Shot.* Dr. Oz Show. Clip. January 11, 2013. https://youtu.be/cr4RImZVHiY.

[131] kale120903. *Piers Morgan Got Sick Not Once but Twice after Flu Shot.* Clip. nd. https://youtu.be/3ups38aHGBE

[132] *8 Things to Learn about Ebola from Nancy Snyderman's Live Facebook Chat.* Today. Jul. 31, 2014. http://www.today.com/health/8-things-learn-about-ebola-dr-nancy-snydermans-live-facebook-1D80001924

[133] Kaplan, Don. *Dr. Nancy Snyderman departs NBC News, announces plan to teach at major medical school.* NY Daily News. March 12, 2015.
http://www.nydailynews.com/entertainment/tv/dr-nancy-snyderman-fired-nbc-news-article-1.2147479.

[134] Ziv, Stav. *NBC's Nancy Snyderman Breaks Ebola Quarantine, Apologizes.* Newsweek. October 14, 2014.
http://www.newsweek.com/nbcs-nancy-snyderman-breaks-ebola-quarantine-apologizes-277380.

[135] NPR. *Zero Ebola Cases in Sierra Leone, as Epidemic Peters Out.* Aug 20, 2015.
http://www.npr.org/sections/goatsandsoda/2015/08/20/432881760/zero-ebola-cases-reported-in-sierra-leone-as-epidemic-peters-out

[136] *Every Week Hundreds of People Get Hepatitis B.* NY Department of Health. October, 2012.
https://www.health.ny.gov/publications/2340/

[137] Gallagher, C. & Goodman, M.S. *Hepatitis B Vaccine of Male Neonates and Autism Diagnosis* NHIS 1992-2002 Journal of Toxicology and Environmental Health. 2010;73(24):1665-77.
https://www.ncbi.nlm.nih.gov/pubmed/21058170.

[138] Frontline. "The Vaccine War." April 27, 2010.
http://www.pbs.org/wgbh/pages/frontline/vaccines/interviews/offit.html

[139] http://www.merriam-webster.com/dictionary/Occam's%20razor

[140] Mayo Clinic. *Guilllain-Barre Syndrome.* nd.
http://www.mayoclinic.org/diseases-conditions/guillain-barre-syndrome/basics/definition/con-20025832.

[141] CDC. *Contraindications and Precautions in Commonly Used Vaccines in Adults* CDC. 2016. http://www.cdc.gov/vaccines/schedules/hcp/imz/adult-contraindications.html

[142] ttp://www.whale.to/m/haley.html

[143] Peebles, J.M. *Compulsory Vaccination*. Los Angeles: Peebles Publishing Company, 1913. http://www.whale.to/c/peebles1.pdf.

[144] Atkinson, Sheryl. *Leading Doctor. Vaccines-Autism Worth Study*. CBS News. May 12, 2008. http://www.cbsnews.com/news/leading-dr-vaccines-autism-worth-study/

[145] Pearlstein, Joanna. *The Sickeningly Low Vaccination Rates at Silicon Valley Day Care.* Wired. October 11, 2015. https://www.wired.com/2015/02/tech-companies-and-vaccines/

[146] Candyce Estave Interivew of Judy Mikovits https://vimeo.com/146831570

[147] Hewitson L., et. al. *Influence of Pediatric Vaccines on Amygdala Growth and Opioid Ligand Binding in Rhesus Macaque Infants: A Pilot Study.* Acta Neurobiol Exp (Wars). 2010. 2010;70(2):147-64. https://www.ncbi.nlm.nih.gov/pubmed/20628439

[148] Hooker, B. *Measles Mumps Rubella Vaccination Timing in Autism among Young African American Boys; A Reanalysis of the CDC Data.* Translational Neurodegeneration 2014 3:22. https://www.ncbi.nlm.nih.gov/pmc/articles/PMC4183946/

[149] Eisenstein, Mayer. *Don't Vaccinate Before You Educate*. Free Download Website. 2014. https://dreisenstein.leadpages.net/vaccine-law-downloadpage-name/

[150] American Medical Association. *Code of Medical Ethics*. 2016. https://www.ama-assn.org/about-us/code-medical-ethics

[151] CDC. "Tetanus." nd. http://www.cdc.gov/tetanus/about/causes-transmission.html

[152] Aceh Epidemiology Group. *Outbreak of Tetanus Cases Following the Tsunami in Aceh Province, Indonesia.* Global Public Health 2006;1(2):173-7. https://www.ncbi.nlm.nih.gov/pubmed/19153905

[153] CDC. *Epidemiology and Prevention of Vaccine-Preventable Diseases: Tetanus.* nd. http://www.cdc.gov/vaccines/pubs/pinkbook/tetanus.html

[154] Ohlheiser, Abby. *The Tense Standoff between Catholic Bishops and the Kenyan Government over Tetanus Vaccines.* Washington Post. Nov 14, 2014. https://www.washingtonpost.com/news/worldviews/wp/2014/11/14/the-tense-standoff-between-catholic-bishops-and-the-kenyan-government-over-tetanus-vaccines/?utm_term=.2fb648c2fcf2

[155] Talwar, G.P., et. al. *Birth Control Vaccine is on the Horizon for Family Planning.* Ann Med. 1993 Apr; 25(2): 207-12. https://www.ncbi.nlm.nih.gov/pubmed/7683889

[156] Lupus Foundation of America. *Children Born to Mothers with Lupus Might be at Increased Risk of Autism.* Oct 28, 2013. http://www.lupus.org/research-news/entry/children-born-to-mothers-with-lupus-might-be-at-increased-risk-of-autism

[157] Greenlee, John. *Encephalitis.* Merck Manual: Consumer Version. http://www.merckmanuals.com/home/brain,-spinal-cord,-and-nerve-disorders/brain-infections/encephalitis

[158] Kassis I, et.al. *Long Term Motor and Cognitive Effects of Acute Encephalitis.* Pediatrics. 2014 Mar;133(3):e546-52. https://www.ncbi.nlm.nih.gov/pubmed/24534397

[159] Sing, V.K., et.al. *Abnormal Measles Mumps Rubella Antibodies and CNS Autoimmunity in Children with Autism.* Sing VK J Biomedical Science. 2002 Jul-Aug;9(4):359-64. https://www.ncbi.nlm.nih.gov/pubmed/12145534

[160] National Institute of Arthritis and Musculoskeletal and Skin Diseases National Institute of Health. https://www.niams.nih.gov/

[161] Scoenfeld, Y., & Agmon-Levin, N. *ASIA Autoimmune Inflammatory Syndrome Induced by Adjuvants.* J Autoimmun. 2011 Feb; 36(1): 4-8. https://www.ncbi.nlm.nih.gov/pubmed/20708902

[162] Le Houzec, D. *Evolution of Multiple Sclerosis in France Since the Beginning of the Hepatitis B Vaccination.* Immunological Research. 2014; 60(2-3): 219–225. https://www.ncbi.nlm.nih.gov/pubmed/25395338

[163] http://www.nvic.org/CMSTemplates/NVIC/pdf/Live-Virus-Vaccines-and-Vaccine-Shedding.pdfhttp://www.hrsa.gov/vaccinecompensation/adverseeffects.pdf

[164] CDC. *Update: Vaccine Side Effects, Adverse Reactions, Contraindications, and Precautions Recommendations of the Advisory Committee on Immunization Practices (ACIP).* MMWR. September 06, 1996. http://www.cdc.gov/mmwr/preview/mmwrhtml/00046738.htm

[165] Horvath, Karen. *Gastrointestinal Abnormalities in Children with Autistic Disorder*. Journal of Pediatrics. 1999 Nov;135(5):559-63.
https://www.ncbi.nlm.nih.gov/pubmed/10547242.

[166] Division of Toxicology and Environmental Medicine. *Aluminum.* ATSDR. September 2008.
http://www.atsdr.cdc.gov/toxprofiles/tp22-c1-b.pdf

[167] Shaw, C., Tomljenovic, L. *Mechanisms of Aluminum Adjuvant Toxicity and Autoimmunity in Pediatric Populations*. Shaw C Lupus. 2012 Feb;21(2):223-30.
https://www.ncbi.nlm.nih.gov/pubmed/22235057

[168] Miller, N. *Aluminum in Vaccines: A Neurological Gamble.* Thinktwice Global Vaccine Institute, 2010.
http://thinktwice.com/aluminum.pdf.

[169] FDA. *Title 21: Food and Drugs.* April 1, 2016.
http://www.accessdata.fda.gov/scripts/cdrh/cfdocs/cfcfr/CFRSearch.cfm?fr=201.323

[170] Miller, N. *Aluminum in Vaccines: A Neurological Gamble.* Thinktwice Global Vaccine Institute, 2010.
http://thinktwice.com/aluminum.pdf

[171] Shaw, C, & Tomljenovic L. Do aluminum vaccine adjuvants contribute to the rising prevalence of autism? J Inorganic Biochemistry. 2011 Nov;105(11):1489-99. 23.
http://www.ncbi.nlm.nih.gov/pubmed/22099159

[172] Fewtrell M.S., et. al. *Aluminum Exposure from Parenteral Nutrition in Preterm Infants: Bone Health at 15-year Follow-Up*. Pediatrics. 2009 Dec;124(6):1709.
https://www.ncbi.nlm.nih.gov/pubmed/19858156

[173] Cenziper, D. *A Disputed Diagnosis Imprisons Parents, Prosecutors Build Murder Cases on Disputed Shaken Baby Syndrome Diagnosis.* Washington Post. March 20, 2015. https://www.washingtonpost.com/graphics/investigations/shaken-baby-syndrome/

[174] Ayoub, D., et. al. *A Critical Review of the Classic Metaphyseal Lesion: Traumatic or Metabolic.* AJR Am J Roentgenol. 2014 Jan;202(1):185-96. https://www.ncbi.nlm.nih.gov/pubmed/24370143.

[175] Vissner, W.J. &Van de Vyver, F.L. *Aluminum Induced Osteocalcin in Severe Chronic Renal Failure.* Visser WJ Clin Nephrol. 1985;24 Suppl 1:S30-6. https://www.ncbi.nlm.nih.gov/pubmed/3915958.

[176] Sears, R. *Aluminum Information from The Vaccine Book.* Ask Dr. Sears Website. nd. http://www.askdrsears.com/topics/health-concerns/vaccines/vaccine-faqs

[177] Fraser, H. *The Peanut Allergy Epidemic: What's Causing It and How to Stop It.* NY: Skyhorse, 2011.

[178] Pichichero, M.E., et. al. *Mercury Concentrations and Metabolism in Infants Receiving Vaccines Containing Thimerosal.* Lancet. 2002 Nov 30;360(9347):1737-41. https://www.ncbi.nlm.nih.gov/pubmed/12480426

[179] Burbacher, T., et. al. *Comparison of Blood Brain Mercury Levels in Infant Levels in Infant Monkeys Exposed to Methyl Mercury or Vaccines Containing Thimerosal.* Environmental Health Perspectives. 2005 Aug;113(8):1015-21. https://www.ncbi.nlm.nih.gov/pubmed/16079072

[180] Bernard, S., et. al. *Autism, a Novel Form of Mercury Poisoning.* Medical Hypotheses; 2001. 56(4), 462-471.
http://www.safeminds.org/wp-content/uploads/2013/04/Bernard-et-al-2001.pdf

[181] Robert Kennedy Jr. Speech. Autism One Conference, 2013

[182] Schubert J., Riley E.J., & Tyler S.A. *Combined Effects in Toxicology. A Rapid Systematic Testing Procedure: Cadmium, Mercury, and Lead.* Toxicol Environ Health 1978;4(5/6):763-776.
https://www.ncbi.nlm.nih.gov/pubmed/731728

[183] CDC. *Thimerosal in Vaccines.* nd.
http://www.cdc.gov/vaccinesafety/concerns/thimerosal/.

[184] *Highlights of Prescribing Information: Flulaval.* FDA. nd.
http://www.fda.gov/downloads/BiologicsBloodVaccines/Vaccines/ApprovedProducts/UCM112904.pdf

[185] Eli Lilly and Company. *Thimerosal.* December 22, 1999.
http://www.putchildrenfirst.org/media/1.13.pdf

[186] Binkley, Collin. *Scientists Say Fetal Tissue Remains Essential for Vaccines and Developing Treatments.* PBS News Hour. August 11, 2015.
http://www.pbs.org/newshour/rundown/medical-researchers-say-fetal-tissue-remains-essential/

[187] CDC. *Appendix B: Vaccine Excipient and Media Summary, Excipients Included in the US, Vaccine by Vaccine.* April, 2015.
http://www.cdc.gov/VACCINEs/pubs/pinkbook/downloads/appendices/B/excipient-table-2.pdf

[188] Gajdova, M., et.al. *Delayed Effects of Neonatal Exposure to Tween 80 on Female Reproductive Organs in Rats.* Food Chem Toxicology. 1993 Mar;31(3):183-90.
https://www.ncbi.nlm.nih.gov/pubmed/8473002

[189] Siniscalo, D.. et. al. *The Invitro GcMAF Effects on Enndocannabanoid System Transcriptonics, Receptor Formation and Cell Activity on Autism Derived Microphages.* J Journal of Neuroinflammation. 2014 Apr 17;11:78.
https://www.ncbi.nlm.nih.gov/pmc/articles/PMC3996516/

[190] Yamamoto, N. *Deglycoslation of Serum Vitamin D Binding Protein Leads to Immuno Suppression in Cancer Patients.* Cancer Research. 1996 Jun 15;56(12):2827-31.
https://www.ncbi.nlm.nih.gov/pubmed/8665521?dopt=Abstract

[191] *Eczema Vaccinatum.* Pediatrics. August 1958, 2(2).

[192] *Highlights of Prescribing Information: Flumist.* FDA. nd.
http://www.fda.gov/downloads/BiologicsBloodVaccines/Vaccines/ApprovedProducts/UCM294307.pdf

[193] *Important Safety Information: FluMist.Quadrivalent.* Company Website.
https://www.flumistquadrivalent.com/hcp/live-attenuated-vaccine

[194] *Vaccine Information Statement: Influenza (Flu) Vaccine (Live, Intranasal). What You Need to Know.* August 7, 2015.
http://www.cdc.gov/vaccines/hcp/vis/vis-statements/flulive.pdf

[195] Warfel, J.M., Zimmerman, L.I., Merkel, T.J. *Acellular Pertussis Vaccines Protect Against Disease but Fail to Prevent Infection and Transmission in a Nonhuman Primate Model*. Proc. Natl. Acad. Science USA. 2014 Jan 14;111(2):787-92.
http://www.ncbi.nlm.nih.gov/pubmed/24277828

[196] CDC. *For Parents: Vaccines for Your Children*. December 13, 2013.
http://www.cdc.gov/vaccines/parents/infographics/protect-babies-from-whooping-cough.html

[197] Choi, Gloria, The Maternal Interleukin-17a A Pathway in Mice promotes Autism Like Phenotypes in Offspring January 28, 2016 Science.
http://science.sciencemag.org/content/early/2016/01/27/science.aad0314

[198] Infanrix package Insert
https://www.fda.gov/downloads/BiologicsBloodVaccines/Vaccines/ApprovedProducts/UCM124514.pdf

[199] https://twitter.com/hillaryclinton/status/562456798020386l8116?lang=en

[200] Maher, B. *Anti-Pharma Rant*. September 28, 2007.
https://youtu.be/rHXXTCc-IVg

[201] Benjamin, M. *UPI Investigates The Vaccine Conflict*. July 21, 2003. UPI.com. http://www.upi.com/UPI-Investigates-The-vaccine-conflict/44221058841736/

[202] *Announcement of CDC Name Change*. October 3, 1992. 41(43); 829-830.
http://www.cdc.gov/mmwr/preview/mmwrhtml/00017962.htm

[203] *Pfizer Exec: Company Approved of Off Label Use of Bextra Promotion.* Jim Edwards Money Watch. CBS News. June 22, 2009. http://www.cbsnews.com/news/pfizer-exec-company-approved-of-off-label-bextra-promotion/

[204] Ornstein, C., et. al. *Dollars for Docs: How Industry Dollars Reach your Doctors.* Propublica. March 17, 2016. https://projects.propublica.org/docdollars/

[205] Narayana, K.P. *Controversial Vaccine Studies: Why is the Bill and Melinda Gates Foundation Under Fire from the Critics in India.* Economic Times. August 31, 2014. http://articles.economictimes.indiatimes.com/2014-08-31/news/53413161_1_hpv-vaccine-cervarix-human-papilloma-virus

[206] Sheridan, K. *Forgotten Freezer Held Much More than Smallpox.* Yahoo News. July 16, 2014. https://www.yahoo.com/news/forgotten-freezer-held-much-more-smallpox-205440611.html?ref=gs

[207] Packel, D. *FCA claims on Merck Mumps Vaccine to Advance.* Law360 Antitrust. Sept 5, 2014. http://www.law360.com/articles/574389/antitrust-fca-claims-on-merck-mumps-vaccine-to-advance

[208] Raymond, J. *Harvard Mumps Outbreak Continues, but Commencement Will Go On.* NBC News. May 17, 2016. http://www.nbcnews.com/feature/college-game-plan/harvard-mumps-outbreak-continues-commencement-will-go-n575526

[209] Rogers, G. *Scientist who Faked AIDS Research Indicted.* USA Today. June 19, 2014. http://www.usatoday.com/story/news/nation/2014/06/19/fake-aids-research/10899589/

[210] *Former Iowa State Researcher Sentenced for Making False Statements.* Press Release. US Attorney's Office, Southern District of Iowa. July 1, 2015. https://www.justice.gov/usao-sdia/pr/former-iowa-state-researcher-sentenced-making-false-statements

[211] Soltis, A. *Professor Admits Faking AIDS Vaccines to Get 19m in Grants.* NY Post. December 26, 2013. http://nypost.com/2013/12/26/professor-admits-faking-aids-vaccine-to-get-19m-in-grants/

[212] Sheller, Ludwig & Badey. Submission for January 31, 2001 Advisory Committee Meeting. Private letter. January 24, 2001. http://www.fda.gov/ohrms/dockets/ac/01/briefing/3680b2_21.pdf

[213] Nigrovic, L.E. *The Lyme Vaccine: A Cautionary Tale.* Epidemiology and Infection. 2007 Jan; 135(1): 1–8. https://www.ncbi.nlm.nih.gov/pmc/articles/PMC2870557/

[214] *Fugitive Profiles.* Office of Inspector General. nd. https://oig.hhs.gov/fraud/fugitives/profiles.asp

[215] *Three Years and Counting for Failure to Prosecute Poul Thorsen.* Safeminds.org Blog. April 14, 2014. http://www.safeminds.org/blog/2014/04/14/three-years-counting-failure-prosecute-poul-thorsen/

[216] Madsen, K. et. al. *Thimerosal and the Incidence of Autism: Negative Ecological Evidence from Danish Population-Based Data.* Pediatrics. 2003: 112(3). http://pediatrics.aappublications.org/content/112/3/604

[217] Toni. *Vaccine researcher Flees with $2M.* Laleva.org Blog. Mar 11, 2010. http://www.laleva.org/eng/2010/03/nbc_11_atlanta_reports_vaccine_researcher_flees_with_2m.html

[218] *Background Report: Poul Thorsen MD PhD.* CA: SafeMinds.org. November 2012. http://www.safeminds.org/wp-content/uploads/2015/04/Thorsen-Background-Report-Nov-2012.pdf

[219] Rep. *Bill Posey Calling for an Investigation of the CDC's MMR Research Fraud.* Cable News Blog. July 29, 2015.http://www.c-span.org/video/?c4546421/rep-bill-posey-calling-investigation-cdcs-mmr-reasearch-fraud

[220] Morgan Verkamp LLC. *Statement of William W Thompson PhD: Regarding the 2004 article examining the possibility of a relationship between MMR Vaccine and autism.* MorganVerkamp Website. August 27, 2014. https://morganverkamp.com/statement-of-william-w-thompson-ph-d-regarding-the-2004-article-examining-the-possibility-of-a-relationship-between-mmr-vaccine-and-autism/

[221] Hooker, B. *Measles Mump Rubella timing and autism among young African American Boys: A Reanalysis of CDC Data.* Translational Neurodegeneration. 2014 3(16). http://translationalneurodegeneration.biomedcentral.com/articles/10.1186/2047-9158-3-16

[222] Barry, K. *Vaccine Whistleblower: Exposing Autism Research Fraud at the CDC.* NY: Skyhorse, 2015.

[223] *"Isolated" autism – Your child?* nd. No publication attribution. https://vimeo.com/user5503203/review/108522744/186711a23b

[224] *Tic and Repetitive Behavior Disorder Clinic*. Johns Hopkins Hospital Website. nd. http://www.hopkinsmedicine.org/psychiatry/specialty_areas/child_adolescent/patient_information/outpatient/broadway_campus/tics.html

[225] Barry, K. *Vaccine Whistleblower: Exposing Autism Research Fraud at the CDC*. NY: Skyhorse, 2015. p. 37.

[226] Timmerman, L *Merck's Julie Gerberding, Former CDC director on the future of vaccines*, Xconomy. June 24, 2011. http://www.xconomy.com/national/2011/06/24/mercks-julie-gerberding-former-cdc-director-on-the-future-of-vaccines/

[227] *Unraveling the Mysteries of Autism.* Transcript. Housecall with Sanjay Gupta. March 8, 2008 CNN. http://transcripts.cnn.com/TRANSCRIPTS/0803/29/hcsg.01.html

[228] *Robert F Kennedy Jr. The truth about vaccine science Robert F Kennedy Jr. May 19, 2015.*

[229] Offit, P. *Dr. Offit's Abbreviated Resume.* Paul Offit's Website. 2015. http://paul-offit.com/about/

[230] Wakefield, A., et.al. *Illeal Lymphoid Nodular Hyperplasia Nonspecific Colitis and Pervasive Developmental Disorder in Children.* Lancet (Retracted) 1998; 351(9103), 637-641. http://www.thelancet.com/journals/lancet/article/PIIS0140-6736(97)11096-0/abstract

[231] Taylor, G. *"No Evidence of Any Link."* Adventures in Autism Blog. June 14, 2007. http://adventuresinautism.blogspot.co.uk/2007/06/no-evidence-of-any-link.html

[232] Berezow, A. *Vaccine Autism Researcher Should Be Indicted.* CNN. Jan 14, 2011.
http://www.cnn.com/2011/OPINION/01/14/berezow.autism.vaccine.link/

[233] Elizabeth Birt Center for Autism Law and Advocacy. *Co-Author of Lancet MMR-Autism Study Exonerated on all charges of professional misconduct.* nd.
https://www.ebcala.org/areas-of-law/vaccine-law/co-author-of-lancet-mmr-autism-study-exonerated-on-all-charges-of-professional-misconduct

[234] *British Court Throws out Conviction of Autism/Vaccine MD: Andrew Wakefield Set for Full Exoneration Sues British Medical Journal.* Health Impact News. December 8, 2016.
https://healthimpactnews.com/2012/british-court-throws-out-conviction-of-autismvaccine-md-andrew-wakefields-co-author-completely-exonerated/

Part 5: Friendly Advice on Detoxification, Diets, and IEP Success

[235] American Heritage Dictionary.

[236] *Constipation Treatment.* Family Medicine Program University of Alabama. nd.
http://www.fammed.usouthal.edu/Guides&JobAids/handouts/Constipation.pdf

[237] http://www.endfatigue.com/tools-support/vitamin-c-flush.html

[238] *Magnesium.* WebMD. nd.
http://www.webmd.com/vitamins-supplements/ingredientmono-998-

[239] Safety and Efficacy of the Milk and Molasses Enema in the Emergency Department. Gary M Vike MD Medscape February 24, 2017
http://www.medscape.com/viewarticle/845939

[240] *Q&A: Sudden Symptoms are First Sign of PANS and PANDAS.* Stanford Children's Health. July 8, 2015.
http://healthier.stanfordchildrens.org/q-sudden-symptoms-first-sign-pans-pandas/

[241] Ibid.

[242] Fang, B.J., et.al. *Disturbed Sleep: Linking Allergic Rhinitis, Mood and Suicidal Behavior.* Frontiers in Bioscience. 2010 2; 30-46.
http://europepmc.org/abstract/med/20036927

[243] Shattock, P., & Whitely, P. *Biochemical Aspects of Autism Spectrum Disorders: Updating the Opiate Excess Theory and Presenting New Opportunities for Biomedical Intervention.* Expert Opinions in Therapeutic Targets. 2002 Apr;6(2):175-83. https://www.ncbi.nlm.nih.gov/pubmed/12223079

[244] *Dermatitis Herpetiformis.* Medline Plus. NIH. nd.
https://www.nlm.nih.gov/medlineplus/ency/article/001480.htm

[245] Grimm, L. *12 Common Intestinal Parasites.* Medscape. July 15, 2015.
http://reference.medscape.com/features/slideshow/intestinal-parasites

[246] *Parasite Alert: 3 Signs to Watch Out For!* Body Ecology. Advertisement Blog.
http://bodyecology.com/articles/parasite-alert

[247] Clark, H. *Dr. Hulda Clark Herbal Parasite Cleanse for Beginners.* Blog: DrClark.net. 2016.
http://www.drclark.net/cleanses/beginners/herbal-parasite-cleanse/parasite-chart-for-adults

[248] 22 Cater, R.E. Chronic Intestinal Candidiasis is a possible Etiological factor in Chronic Fatigue Syndrome. Medical Hypothesis. 1995 Jun;44(6):507-15.
https://www.ncbi.nlm.nih.gov/pubmed/7476598

Made in the USA
Lexington, KY
22 March 2017